Some Dietary Quotes

'Tis not her coldness, father, That chills my labouring breast;
It's that confounded cucumber I've ate and can't digest.
Richard Harris Barham: *The Confession*

Better is a dinner of herbs where love is, than a stalled ox and hatred there-
with. *Proverbs* (ch. XV, v. 17)

The stomach carries the heart, and not the heart the stomach.
[Spanish, *Tripas llevan corazon, que no corazon tripas.*]
Miguel de Cervantes Saavedra: *Don Quixote* (ch. II, 47)

History is apt to judge harshly those who sacrifice tomorrow for today.
Harold MacMillan

Thou shouldst eat to live; not live to eat.
[Latin, *Esse oportet ut vivas, non vivere ut edas.*]
Cicero: *Rhetoricorum Ad C. Herennium* (IV, 7)

We think fast food is equivalent to pornography, nutritionally speaking.
Steve Elbert

We are all dietetic sinners; only a small percent of what we eat nourishes us;
the balance goes to waste and loss of energy.   Sir William Osler

Other books by Keith Scott-Mumby

The Food Allergy Plan 1985
Allergies: What Everyone Should Know 1986
The Allergy Handbook 1988
The Poisoned Tree 1990
Thorson's Complete Guide to Food Allergy and Environmental Illness 1994
Virtual Medicine 1999
To Fly Without Wings 2003

DIET WISE

Toxic Foods Are Common and Cause
a Lot of Harm. Everyone is Different.
Find Out Yours.

By
Dr. Keith Scott-Mumby
MB ChB, MD, PhD, FCRP *(Colombo)*

Mother Whale Inc.
P.O. Box 19452, Reno,
NV 89511
USA

Distributors:
Please contact
Brigham Distributors,
110 S. 800 W. Brigham City,
UT 84302
Tel: 435 723 6611

10 9 8 7 6 5

ISBN-13: 978-0-9838784-1-4
ISBN-10: 0-9838784

Printed in USA by
Bang Printing, 3323 Oak St, Brainerd, MN 56401
www.bangprinting.com

Cover design by Andy Reifert (www.brightbulbideas.com)

Graphics by Oliver Scott-Mumby (www.citizenmoose.com)

Layout by Dragos Balasoiu (contact@dragosb.com)

Contents

This book is dedicated to my second wife Vivien,
who has made my life a joy.

ACKNOWLEDGMENTS

I'd like to say thank you to all those who helped in the writing of this book. That includes over 10,000 patients and their suffering families: too many to mention by name, even if I had encyclopedic recall.

Thanks also to my great mentors Theron Randolph, MD, William Rea MD, Richard Mackarness MD, Doris Rapp MD, Prof. Jonathan Brostoff and those who went before but I never met: Herbert Rinkel, Michael Zeller and Warren T. Vaughan Sr.

Thanks also to my editor Karen McChrystal, whose expertise and patience has enabled this project to go forward smoothly.

Toxic Foods: The Original Detox Diet

Over thirty years ago a handful of doctors, myself among them, began working with what is today called a "detox" diet. We discovered that foods could indeed be very toxic to an individual.

I'm not talking here about fast foods and manufactured junk—or known poisonous plants—which are bad for everyone. I'm talking here about intolerance of everyday foods; good foods; whole foods even! It was an individual, idiosyncratic thing.

We had little notion then of the nature of minor genetic variants in a person's genome causing metabolic food intolerance. We thought in terms of "food allergy". It was a contentious idea. Colleagues argued; lines were drawn; a furious battle broke out. Ultimately patients were the losers. For while orthodox doctors were busily arguing that food could not cause allergies on anything like the scale we were seeing, that hubris distracted them from grasping the enormous importance of what we pioneers were seeing in a clinical practice.

Over the years, and on seeing tens of thousands of patients, I observed removing toxic foods from a person's diet could cure a vast number of serious illnesses including – but not limited to - eczema, dermatitis, migraine, colitis, high blood pressure, obesity, anorexia, depression and alcoholism, as well as a whole host of minor complaints, such as headaches, bellyaches, joint pains, low moods, abdominal boating, catarrh, difficulty waking in the morning, overweight, palpitations, panic attacks, inability to concentrate (wooly brain), lack of libido and general fatigue.

Even cancer, schizophrenia and mental cases did better.

Getting rid of toxic foods also resulted in looking great, feeling good, losing lots of weight without needing to feel hungry, getting rid of age spots and wrinkles, all of which made a person look a dozen years younger and brought boundless zestful energy

Yet it was relatively easy to do. Once properly identified, avoiding a few toxic foods was far preferable to a life of suffering or chronic pill taking.

Patients recovered and were rightly grateful and joyful. It was a whole new enjoyable way of life: fresh, healthy, free and exciting.

Even breaking the taboo foods once in a while did not result in a relapse for most. I used to liken this subject to a game and explain to patients there are rules; simple rules to be sure. But like any game, if you didn't know the rules, you had little chance of winning!

I'm going to teach you all the rules. I'll explain everything you need to know right here in these pages, how to do it for yourself, without medical help or any specialist knowledge. It may be the only diet book you will ever need. Sounds unbelievable?

Well, just keep reading. It's all here. But don't skip. This diet is totally different from anything you have read before. It's basically a **Custom Fit Diet**. The reason I say that will become clear as we go along. You need to understand how it works, and why. The early chapters lay down important ground work for success and you will learn things your doctor probably doesn't even know about, much less discuss with you. Later we get to how you carry out the actual steps.

Be patient. This is a whole revolution we're talking here; it's a lot to absorb.

I was taught these little-known secrets by earlier pioneers and got miraculous results which catapulted me into media fame around the world. For the first time in my career as a physician I began to see real recoveries, real cures. I saw fewer patients, because it takes longer using this route, but I made more sincere and lasting friends among my patients than I ever did in the bad old days of pill pushing. In fact for almost forty years I have hardly ever prescribed a pharmaceutical drug! Those who want them can always get them from eager doctors, whose approach disease is dominated by the pseudo-science of Big Pharma.

I have become a teacher in turn and realize that what I have learned over the decades is a considerable body of diet wisdom that is vital for everyone. This book summarizes most of what I know and is intended for those who want to take control of their own health and learn the whys and wherefores of body function and nutritional science.

Pills for Everything

Chronic pill-popping is one of the hallmarks of our age. Conventional medicine has sold us on the idea that there is a chemical for everything, from bereavement to schizophrenia, panic attacks to asthma, heartburn to malignant tumors. This is the mentality which insists that depression is just a Prozac-deficiency; this is the floundering science that says the answer to side-effects from drugs is more drugs.

But my standpoint is that any chronic medication is by definition a failure: it doesn't cure. If it did, there would be no need to continue taking it! The best that this kind of therapy can do is treat symptoms. Even then, it only masks them, because it is not based on solving the cause of the problem but on suppressing the results. This has been likened to covering up the oil warning light on your automobile. The symptom (red light) goes away but the oil pressure remains too low and your automobile will die young. If only my colleagues understood this in full.

I'd like to offer my own unique definition of a successful cure, which is brutal and short: *no symptoms, no treatment.* If the condition needs repeated treatment, even holistic remedies, to keep symptoms at bay, it isn't a cure. No disease, no requirement for treatment – that's a cure! The only way you are going to get that happy result is to call up Mother Nature. Without her you will cure nothing, heal nothing, solve nothing.

Stay well and live long

You don't need to be sick to benefit from this plan. If you consider yourself fit and well, follow these steps and stay well for the rest of your life! We now know that what you eat is a crucial and personal thing; what you eat interacts with your genes and not every food is right for your genetic make up. You'll probably live longer if you customize your diet and figure out which foods are best for you. That's what this book is about. It's the *crucial* aspect of this book.

But the truth is that most of us are not really as healthy as we should be. Maybe you don't admit to serious symptoms; but are you bounding with abundant energy, radiantly happy and fulfilled in all aspects of your life? If not, you are not truly in a state of wellness. That's something else my conventional colleagues have sold to everybody: that health is merely the absence of disease. Not good enough. A positive sense of well being and plenty of energy available whenever needed is what should be regarded as optimum health. That's real vitality.

Maybe you had it as a child and have lost it. Maybe you never felt that good, in which case you have something delightful to discover about healthy living: it feels great – like being in love, getting a big raise or promotion, publishing your first novel and winning the state lottery, all rolled into one! When would be a good time to rediscover the best feelings of your life, to regain lost youth and beat off those annoying little signals of less-than-perfect health?

If not now, when?

Eating dangerously

The title for this section comes from a book published in 1976 by a UK physician named Richard Mackarness (published in Britain as *Not all in the Mind*). It became something of a classic and many years later I was asked to write a foreword by the publishers, Thorsons, an imprint of Harper Collins. I compared it to other radical and seminal alternative books, such as *Silent Spring* by Rachel Carson and *Small is Beautiful* by Ernest Schumacher.

Mackarness' message was that food can make you ill – sometimes very ill. I read *Eating Dangerously* a few years after it was published and it changed my career utterly and led to the happiest days of my life. It was certainly contentious and challenging reading. But instead of dismissing it as nonsense, which most trained doctors did, I determined to find out for myself. I started putting patients on a suggested eating plan, avoiding the common danger foods, and they began to get well, suddenly and dramatically. Aches and pains vanished, chronic disease suddenly went away, people felt better, looked younger and lost weight easily and permanently. Many stopped their medication.

Make no mistake, food can hurt you. In fact it can make your life hell. I'm talking not just about junk food – a common misconception – but good whole food: milk, eggs, wholegrain wheat, fruit and so on. You've been told these foods are healthy, and no doubt, good for you. But I have a different message for you: supposedly healthy natural foods can make some individuals very ill. I have had thousands of patients whose lives were being ruined by eating wholesome foods that they personally did not tolerate but were unaware where the trouble was coming from.

This goes beyond mere food allergy. You might think that allergy to food is rare and has nothing to do with you (you would be mistaken). But it has emerged recently at the cutting edge of science that our genes, which dictate so much of our health also control our food tolerances. A food which is right for one person may be disastrous in the metabolic pathways of another – a modern genetics version of Lucretius' old saw: "One man's meat is another man's poison." The important point for the moment is not why it happens; the critical element is that it can happen with any food, any individual. Avoiding these foods is the key to a long and healthy life.

The trouble is you may not be aware that foods are affecting you in this way. We talk of a hidden allergy or masked allergy to food. This mechanism will be explained in due course but, as the name suggests, it may not be obvious at all where the problem is coming from. Hidden allergies or genetic intolerance can occur to foods eaten frequently, even daily, and yet remain undetected. Curiously, a person may even become addicted to his or her incompatible foods. He or she likes the very thing that is causing the problem.

The first "food allergy" plan

In 1985 I published my own *Food Allergy Plan* (the foundation of this book). Theron Randolph MD, the doyen and founder of this discipline, described it as the best book of its kind in the world. Sales started quietly, because in those days most people were unaware they needed it! Patients with migraine would suppose they had migraine, not food allergy, and so buy a book on migraine (which explained all the drug therapies and how hopeless it was); same with arthritis and scores of other conditions, which in fact are comonly due to toxic food reactions, as we shall see.

Gradually, pushing through, and winning over the public, I found larger and larger audiences willing to listen to the message that what you eat can make you seriously ill. By the mid-80s the media were full of it. Food allergy and intolerance had arrived and I was one of the chief voices saying that it was very common. In fact it is almost universal. Food can be quite toxic.

Nowadays those of us out in front, looking for answers, have begun to realize the genetic incompatibility with foods is at least as important as the allergy phenomenon. Our DNA controls the performance of numerous metabolic pathways and that in turn regulates how we deal with substances introduced into our bodies. Foodstuffs, of course, are nothing more than a conglomerate of chemicals (with a little life energy thrown in!). The emerging new science of nutritional genomics, as it is called, is telling us that the old paradigm in which "bad" foods gave you heart disease or cancer unless "good" genes intervened to protect you is too simplistic and wide of the mark. New research suggests a continual interaction between foods and health, in which certain foods are found to enhance or suppress the action of genes, some of which are protective and some of which may be very harmful.

That means you can regulate your own genes by what you eat, helping them or blocking them. It's all very new and shocking to a body of science that is steeped in the belief that DNA is the inviolate blueprint of our lives but the truth is clear and becoming clearer every day. There is no logic in the search for a universally healthy diet and those authors who proclaim they have one are misleading you. Forget the Atkins Diet, The Perricone Promise, the South Beach Diet or any other pre-determined diet. Even William Wollcott's metabolic typing diet is erroneous in supposing we can all be fitted into just three metabolic types. There are as many unique individual correct diets as there are combinations of genes – and that's almost infinite! Note: this same principle applies if you are using the Gerson Diet or other non-customized diet for cancer control.

This is exactly what I tried to tell the world over 20 years ago with my first book, *The Food Allergy Plan,* but the world was not yet ready and we didn't have the genetic incompatibility model to fill in the gaps where the allergy model didn't suffice. The scientific truth, as you will learn, is that each and every one of us has to discover his or her own personal safe diet. To work out yours you will need to become *diet wise*, exactly as I have described in these pages.

How to live one hundred years

True life examples, I have always felt, enhance understanding and are easier to remember. Here is an historic tale, from Italy.

The central character was a Venetian nobleman called Luigi Cornaro. He was born in 1467, which makes him a contemporary of Michelangelo Buonarotti and Leonarado da Vinci, who were busy, along with numerous others, creating their world-shaking art in Florence as part of the great *Renaissance* (literally rebirth).

Cornaro started his own shift of consciousness phenomenon, as we shall see. His was more studied and scientific but none the less visionary for all that. Through the book you now hold his method of rebirth (health and long life) can come true for us all.

A typical nobleman of the day, Cornaro squandered his considerable fortune on high living, especially food and drink. Unfortunately, his constitution was rather weak and he was racked with symptoms, including indigestion and gout, attended by an almost continuous fever and thirst. He was getting steadily worse. Cornaro would probably have died by the age of forty, as most people did in those days.

But he was lucky. One of his physicians told him, in no uncertain terms, that he had better sober up his lifestyle or call the undertakers.

Shocked by the possibility of imminent death, Cornaro decided the smart thing to do was to listen to the doctor's advice (which for once was sound and holistic). He began to experiment and found that he felt better if he ate less and avoided certain foods that seemed to upset his constitution. In fact Cornaro was the first person on record to work out his own detox diet. He was pretty smart and realized that the foods he liked or craved were not necessarily the best for him.

Cornaro found that he did not tolerate fish, pork, melons and other fruits, salad (though he doesn't say what ingredients), rough wines and pastry. Surprisingly, the foods he could tolerate included meats and certain choice wines. He liked an egg, bread and soup.

Eat less and eat right was his basic formula. In his case he was able to tolerate twelve ounces of food daily and fourteen ounces of decent wine. Within a year he was fully healed, zestful and enjoying life. The years rolled by, fifty, sixty, seventy, eighty! Apart from a couple of episodes, he remained well. One setback was a serious coach accident at the age of seventy, which almost cost him his life. Cornaro was dragged from the wreck with many bruises, a dislocated arm and a broken leg. The doctors wanted to bleed him (as if he weren't shocked enough). Cornaro wisely refused and relied on his own diet management formula to restore his damaged limbs.

It worked.

The second near fatality occurred when he broke his diet, at the insistence of concerned relatives. They believed he should fatten himself up, to maintain his strength. As a result of continued nagging he decided to up his rations to fourteen ounces of food a day and sixteen ounces of wine. Within a week he was peevish and quarreling with all comers. By the tenth day he was seized with a violent pain in his side, which lasted over twenty-two hours, before being succeeded by a serous fever, which lasted for thirty-five days. Cornaro abandoned the changes and soon recovered.

In fact he went on to live an exceptionally long and healthy life. At the amazing age of eighty-three he published his first treatise, entitled *The Sure and Certain Method of Attaining a Long and Healthful Life.* The English translation went through numerous editions. He wrote three more pamphlets on the same subject, composed at the ages of eighty-six, ninety-one and ninety-five respectively.

Luigi Cornaro finally died, serene and dignified, at the age of ninety-eight.

What was remarkable about Cornaro's achievement was that he lived in an age when the average life expectancy was under forty years. To live beyond three score years and ten was almost unheard of, never mind reaching two years short of one hundred. Cornaro had clearly made a major discovery in the field of disease and health; you would think the medicos of the day would be won over and want to pass on the good news.

Instead they ignored Cornaro's remarkable diet experiments.

Casebook 1.

Think all this is historic, beyond our era, and irrelevant? Maybe it sounds too extreme. Do you have to be so strict to live to a hundred years? Certainly not. Let me tell you a story from my casebook.

Arthur was in his sixties when he first made contact with me. His health had deteriorated to the point where he was lying in bed over 20 hours a day, with scarcely strength to move. His heart was weak and enlarged and he had been waiting for a suitable donor to come along, to provide a transplant. Having heard about me and some of the sensational cures that I had been getting by just excluding certain toxic foods, he asked for help.

I put him on exactly the same recommended diet program described here in this book. Within two weeks he was starting to feel better. Within a month he was not only able to travel but actually drove himself to my office. By the time we had completed testing for food culprits, it became clear that wheat was his number one enemy. When he tried to re-introduce it, as described on page 126, he collapsed into his earlier debilitated condition.

Arthur's ideal diet required him to avoid wheat and one or two lesser bandit foods, which he did dutifully. His health recovered to the state where he was fitter than men ten years his junior. He never had the heart transplant and will never need one, I'm sure.

The last time I visited him, before I left the UK for good, I saw Arthur in his home. At the age of 78 he had been erecting a large wooden garden shed. Single-handedly, he had cut timbers, drilled and fixed them, and even put on the roof, which required lifting a considerable weight above his head height. This determined man wanted a small workshop and had decided to build his own!

Diet may be the key to aiding recovery

Today, fortunately, there is a growing awareness that correct eating and good health go hand in hand. With the discovery of the phenomenon of food allergies and genetic food intolerance and the recognition of their widespread harmful effects, the door has been opened for the cure of a wide variety of diseases.

It has been estimated that *over half of all illnesses* reported to doctors are caused or worsened by toxic foods, so this condition is not rare. I will share with you cases that suffered from apparently incurable diseases, which nevertheless got well following the path I lay out in this book. Afflictions such as brain damage, heart enlargement and infertility may seem to have nothing to do with what a person eats, yet the patient improved dramatically, doing what I shall be telling you in this book. How can this happen? The important principle is what we call total body load: if you can reduce the body's problems significantly, Nature can often take care of the rest and work an apparently spontaneous healing.

In addition to major named diseases, there is a great deal of minor symptomatology which is not reported at all: everyone considers it 'normal' to have a few aches and pains. Good health is often taken to be the mere absence of disease. Yet abundant energy, well being, clarity of thinking and zest should be your lot. If this isn't the case, then the advice in this book probably applies to you.

Unfortunately, the medical profession as a whole is entrenched in the belief that diet is unimportant, despite the fact that Hippocrates over two thousand years ago stated that no healing could be truly successful without attention being paid to what the patient was eating. Instead, the conventional doctor blunders on, with newer and more dangerous drugs, always ready with the scalpel or chemo, spurred on by more and more obscure laboratory 'investigations' until the patient is lost in a welter of science. One wonders where it will all end, for whereas in any other profession a narrowness of view is nothing more than an infantile and unbecoming failure, in medicine it is a dangerous neglect of duty from which only the patient suffers. A doctor has a certain responsibility to do the best for his or her patient and that means keeping abreast of any area of new knowledge which may help.

Resistance from the medical establishment

Sadly, the history of medicine does not reflect this responsibility: the first users of anesthetics were struck off as frauds; antisepsis was scorned by surgeons who went on operating in their top hats and coat tails; and Dr. Semmelweis of Vienna was abused to the point of suicide for daring to suggest that doctors wash their hands before examining women in childbed, which demonstrably reduced deadly puerperal fever. Nearer our own time, penicillin, arguably the greatest drug of all time, was ignored for years as a discovery when it could have saved *millions* of lives. Even today, homoeopathy, which cures gently by taking into account the whole person as opposed to merely a part, is fought against with blind fury by doctors who have never tried or tested the efficacy of any of its remedies.

You may think I write bitterly about the resistance to this new work, and you are right, of course. I have had my share of scorn and ridicule from colleagues who never once took the trouble to visit my office and see if the work I did was really valid. But what distresses me most is the disparagement and abuse that patients themselves sometimes have to undergo because of their food incompatibilities. So many times I have had before me sad and dispirited human beings who break into tears of relief when they realize that someone, at last, is willing to listen to their problems and *believe* them. As a rule they have been scolded or told they were neurotic and 'imagining' things. Many of them feel they are a burden to their family doctor when, in some cases, the opposite seems to be true.

I know from the fact that every time I speak on the radio or one of our cases is featured in the press we are deluged with calls that very many people are anxious for help and *don't know where to get it*. That is why this book came to be written. If your own doctor refuses to help, there is little you can do except try to sort things out for yourself. Perhaps this do-it-yourself volume will enable you to do just that. I make no claims to breakthrough discoveries in the field of allergies, but the method which follows is my own, developed over a quarter of a century, and is offered freely to whomever is in need of it.

Within weeks, or even days, you could be free of a chronic or lifelong affliction. Without exaggeration, the lame can walk again, the respiratory cripple can breathe, the sickly and weak become strong, pain and misery diminish to but a memory. It really is a miracle: hundreds of thousands of cases from all over the world attest to it.

Now you too can become truly *diet wise.*

2

Could a Toxic Food
Be Spoiling Your Life?

Adoctor friend of mine, who regarded himself as being in perfect health, did some experimental testing on himself to discover whether he had any food intolerances. He uncovered an allergy to wheat and, as a further test, he omitted wheat from his diet. To his surprise he no longer felt tired at the end of a busy day and woke in the morning with a feeling of exhilaration instead of his usual dread of a heavy day's work. The doctor suddenly realized that his perfect health was far from being as good as it could be.

When bread, which is usually regarded as the staff of life, disagrees with you, and you are an unsuspecting victim of what is happening as a consequence, you can come to regard health as a mere absence of disease. This is not good enough. A positive sense of well being with plenty of energy always ready for use is what should be regarded as normal health.

An allergy to the food you are eating every day can take the edge off your enjoyment of life, can cause you to feel under the weather without anything definite to complain about or can actually be the cause of severe inexplicable illness. But the vast majority of people do not know that this is what is happening to their bodies and state of mind. They simply accept that mystery symptoms which come and go are just normal.

A huge amount of pathology and suffering, from bellyaches, to strange and inappropriate moods, even violence, is dismissed, even by doctors, as just one of those things. But that's ignorance, not science. From the early 80s onwards I made it my business to begin to educate the public about the phenomenon of individual food toxicity, including food allergy and intolerance.

How can you have a hidden allergy or food incompatibility?

It is usual to think of food allergy in terms of the type of illness which results from an allergy to nuts, strawberries or shellfish. These foods, however, are not eaten on a day to day basis, and the violence of the reaction when encountered leaves little opportunity for the source of the illness to remain unsuspected.

But there is an entirely different clinical picture when the food to which you are allergic is a staple item of your diet that you eat every day of your life, perhaps several times each day. Under these circumstances, the body adapts to the allergic process and the reaction disappears to become a masked allergy. This adaptation of the body may last a lifetime or may become exhausted at any time under stress. When the adaptation by the body is complete there are no symptoms, but if the strain of coping with the allergy wears down the adaptive process then a whole variety of symptoms may break the surface.

At different times in a person's life these breakthrough manifestations of the underlying masked allergy, may present themselves in a wide variety of illnesses.

Let us take a typical life story of a person who is allergic to cow's milk. If bottle-fed as a baby there are considerable feeding difficulties. Baby gets a lot of wind and mother gets many sleepless nights.

There may be a long period with a runny nose, repeated ear troubles, sore throats, constant colds, and tonsils and adenoids get removed. The adaptive process may become complete from time to time and all symptoms may disappear. The allergic patient may enjoy periods of excellent health when nothing appears to be wrong. But it is quite usual for the patient to have growing pains, to be over or under active, showing signs of attention deficit disorder (ADD), suffering troublesome headaches and being highly susceptible to infections, with consequent frequent colds and 'flu-like attacks.

At puberty the patient's story may take a dramatic turn, all symptoms may disappear completely or everything may get worse. When puberty brings trouble it can come in many forms: migraine, asthma, eczema, acne, depression and behavior problems. Even vandalism can suddenly turn on as a result of the masked allergy becoming partially unmasked. In girls all manner of menstrual problems may be a result of an unsuspected allergy to foods or chemicals. It seems as though the body becomes supersensitive to its own hormones and any variation in the hormone balance occurring at puberty, at menstruation, during pregnancy or at the menopause may all cause symptoms of varying degrees. These symptoms may be premenstrual tension, heavy painful periods, absence of periods, sickness in pregnancy, toxemia of pregnancy, depression after confinement and all those unpleasant symptoms commonly associated with change of life.

Bizarre and protean symptoms

The sheer variety and variability of symptoms caused by hidden food allergy and genetic food intolerance is the main reason that the problem was not recognized sooner. Doctors are convinced that all diseases should fit into set describable patterns or syndromes. Any group of symptoms that is not listed and named in their textbooks is therefore not considered a real affliction but something from the patient's imagination. The suspicion of hypochondria rises into the red zone when the patient's complaints keep shifting – headache one week, joint pains another, then bowel trouble, then feeling depressed. Doctors quickly dismiss the patient or send them to see a psychiatrist, with the clear inference 'It's all in your mind.'

The fact is, the condition is one and the same – an allergy to food. It is merely the result of the allergy that shifts. Symptoms can be bizarre, protean and very subjective. [Proteus was a Greek sea god, son of Poseidon (Neptune), who kept changing his form whenever he appeared.] Symptoms can be very bizarre, such as headache every Monday but no other day (onions with Sunday dinner), epilepsy after eating carrots, drunk after eating potatoes or orange and sexual arousal after eating chicken – these are all true cases from my files. Subjective symptoms seems to create even more hostility with physicians, yet patients sometimes have difficulty describing what they feel: I have heard complaints such as "hot water running down the inside of my skin and seeing myself down at the end of a long tunnel," or "On some days I feel like there is a heavy stone inside my abdomen." To a regular doctor these are signs of delusion or psychosomatic illness; to me they are clear indications of brain allergy, or altered perception, a fascinating topic we shall come to later.

Any bodily system can be upset by food allergy or genetic food intolerance and in any one patient one or more systems can be involved. We call this concept 'target organs' or 'shock organs.'

Incidentally, the target system involved can change from one period of life to another.

A child with eczema moves on to asthma, then grows out of asthma and develops stomach ulcers or the irritable bowel syndrome. Stress helps to exhaust the adaptive process of the body and aggravate the symptoms. This often makes it appear as though stress is the cause of the trouble. The patient may have to endure psychotherapy, and when this fails to cure the trouble, drugs may be used to suppress the symptoms.

An inappropriate reaction to food and chemicals seems to guarantee an adverse reaction to the drugs and medicines which may be prescribed to treat the symptoms. The patient tends to get worse and becomes a very difficult case, ending up reacting to almost everything.

In a typical case of masked food allergy the patient may suffer mainly from involvement of the central nervous system. Perhaps the most distressing symptom of all is what has been described by patients as the woolly brain syndrome. An inability to concentrate, confused thinking, memory impairment and a tendency to just sit in an inactive torpor, are all symptoms which cause great distress to a patient who is normally highly intelligent, very industrious and exceptionally competent. Depression is a common and distressing symptom. I have often heard patients with this complaint say that they would kill themselves if they could only bring themselves to do it. Life becomes intolerable.

This state of affairs can put an impossible strain on a marriage. In this condition the person does not wish to be touched and may turn nasty in response to any sort of advance from the marital partner.

These patients often come to be labeled neurotic hypochondriacs and because they cannot explain or understand their own predicament they often come to believe themselves to be insane or going insane. Once these patients are put on drugs and become addicted to drugs the true state of affairs is virtually impossible to untangle and many must be ending their days in mental hospitals.

As I have said already, food can do you a great deal of harm.

Casebook 2.

Recently I received an e-mail from out of the blue from an old patient, called Cliff. He had been surfing the Internet and found my website and written to me, full of the delights of life and exploring the new technology. He is now 88 years old.

Cliff came to see me in 1985, when he was 69 years old, with a tale of woe. All his life he had been sick and debilitated. He suffered frequently from what lay people called "bilious attacks" in those days: headaches and vomiting. Nowadays we would call them migraine attacks or "abdominal migraine" when the stomach is so upset.

Cliff's condition was so bad that on the train ride to the honeymoon destination, he had needed to lie down with his head resting on the lap of his new bride (no, he was not drunk, but certainly reacting to food at the wedding feast, as we shall see).

In 1953 he underwent a partial gastrectomy, on the recommendation of a local professor who had diagnosed a stomach ulcer. It didn't work. Twenty-one years later he was subjected to a vagotomy (severing the important vagus nerve to the gut). Again the procedure didn't work – wrong diagnosis and wrong therapy.

By the time Cliff consulted me, he was so weakened that he had difficulty shaving. He would lather up and then have to rest; then shave a little and would need another rest; and so on. He was a very sick old man and felt ready to die.

Fortunately, this was an easy case – allergic to beef and dairy products. I told him to avoid anything from a cow and he has never looked back. He and his wife Joan (who was also a patient of mine) are a game elderly couple, still actively engaged in church and community work. Both claim that they feel fitter and happier now than at any stage in their lives. In fact Cliff boasts he's healthier today than he was sixty years ago. That's the power of *diet wise* eating.

Joan and Cliff, incidentally, illustrate another point I discovered in my practice. Strongly bonded couples tend to drift in the direction of each other's dietary intolerances! It rather echoes the way females living together tend to adopt similar menstrual cycles.

Everyone has toxic foods (including you!)

The hidden or masked food allergy has often been called the hidden enemy, with good reason. It is extraordinarily common and yet little understood or recognized. It's the real reason why detox diets work.

I'm on record with the BBC as saying that virtually everyone has a food allergy (this was years before recognizing genetic food incompatibility as an alternative phenomenon). One can be allergic to anything, even to vitamin supplements. B vitamins are often synthesized from yeast, vitamin C from corn, vitamin E from wheat germ, and so on… A food allergy or intolerance isn't such a big deal if you are generally well, but it is still very common, if you know the right questions to ask. Nancy Wise of the BBC World Service clearly didn't quite believe me and before interviewing me, she sent a roving microphone onto the streets outside Bush House in London. No one was more surprised than she when eighteen out of twenty people stopped said, "Sure I have an allergy," or words to that effect.

It's a matter of perception. Several of the people interviewed had replies such as "I can't eat celery, it makes my fingers swell," "Bananas give me wind," or "Chocolate gives me a headache." Most of them never thought of these reactions as a food allergy, much less a genetic intolerance to food.

But of course that's exactly what it is.

Tracking down and uncovering of the hidden allergy effect has probably been one of the single most important medical discoveries of the last hundred years, *measured simply in terms of the amount of human suffering now able to be alleviated*. Naturally, public interest is high in this new *safe* approach to healing. Many people who thought they were destined to be ill for life and perhaps had been *told* so by doctors who should know better are waking up to the fact that recovery may be attained merely through eating and drinking differently.

Sometimes it happens by chance; you may know stories of this sort. But it is better to have the knowledge and understanding to make discoveries to order; in that way you can help yourself or your family and friends systematically and effectively. I have written this book with that aim in mind.

The allergy epidemic

Little research has been done in this area and we have no factual data to establish either the prevalence of this condition or its cause. Nevertheless a great deal of circumstantial evidence is available from the histories of patients with proven masked allergies. It is usual to discover that something other than the mother's colostrum (first sticky milk) was the first material to enter the stomach after birth (such as corn syrup in a pacifier). Breast-feeding, it seems, protects against the onset of allergies and helps ensure a competent immune system in the infant. The onset of symptoms is very often triggered by medical treatment. Patients very often recover when additives and pollutants are carefully eliminated from their food and drink.

It would seem that we have what may fairly be called an allergy epidemic started by failure of breast feeding, by pollution of the environment, by the addition of chemicals to our food, air and water and to the injudicious use of drugs and medicines.

There is one further very significant trigger that has swung into view: a recent scientific research paper showed the pronounced effects of childhood vaccination in causing subsequent allergies. Even using conventional criteria for allergy (which I believe misses more than 90%

of the problem), the Japanese study showed that 25.6% of children who received the DPT (triple) vaccine had asthma, whereas only 2.3% of children who had not been vaccinated were troubled. That's a well over ten-fold increase. If studies of all atopic disease (bronchial asthma, allergic rhinitis and atopic dermatitis) were combined, the ratio rises to 56.4%, as against 9.3% in the unvaccinated group (a five-fold increase). In other words *over 50% of kids who are vaccinated end up with allergy problems!* [The effect of DPT and BCG vaccinations on atopic disorders. Yoneyama H, Suzuki M, Fujii K, Odajima Y, Arerugi 2000 Jul;49(7):585-92]

Is the problem hereditary?

This is a question that is often asked, and the answer must be guarded until more exact knowledge becomes available. Certainly the problems do run in families, but that does not point to a gene inheritance *per se*. A problem can run in families without being caused by genes: if parents tend to eat poorly and make themselves ill due to maladaptation to foods, the chances are they will do the same to their offspring. The youngsters will tend to pick up the same cooking and eating pattern and pass it on to *their* children, and so the trend continues. Thus allergies may *appear* to be inherited without actually being so. The picture is further complicated by the fact that a great many babies are now being born with allergies already apparent. In many cases this is due to exposure to allergenic foods *in utero*, but that is not the same as 'inherited' in the exact meaning of the word.

I believe the *tendency* is inherited. Statistics suggest that if one parent is affected by allergies the child has a somewhat higher than fifty per cent chance of being affected also. If both parents are cases, that likelihood rises to about eighty-five per cent – approaching certainty. Exactly *what* those allergies are, however, depends largely on what you come into contact with, *not* on what your parents reacted to; thus if a mother has a milk allergy and avoids milk while pregnant, this is unlikely to become her child's allergy. Similarly, the resultant illness may be different: one parent may have asthma, the other eczema, and yet the child has, say, colitis.

I had one family constellation who were all allergic to wheat, yet the symptoms varied greatly: one had migraines, another skin rashes, the mother had colitis, a child had behavioral disturbance and so on. It was even possible to look back through the generations. The maternal grandfather had schizophrenia. Following the work of Dr. F. C. Dohan, it is possible to suspect that his mental illness was also the result of a severe wheat intolerance.

You will read later about 'target organs' and why there is so much variation from one person to the next, even with the same condition, or more baffling, until you understand the reasons for it even from day to day in the *same person*.

Food toxins

It isn't all about allergies. Intolerance of foods may be simply a reaction to substances contained in the foods, and individual reactions depend on genetic make up. Nature has seen fit to endow a number of plants with the capacity to synthesize substances that are toxic to humans and other animals. Farmers and veterinarians have known for years that animals become sick if they graze on certain types of plant. For example, bulls become enraged if they eat locoweed – 'loco' being Spanish for crazy. Many plant substances are toxic to humans in quite small quantities, including deadly nightshade, acorns and hemlock. Ricin, the toxic principle in castor bean (Ricinus communis), is one of the most poisonous substances known: a minute drop on the tip of a needle was used in an infamous political assassination on the streets of London in 1978: the slaying of Bulgarian dissident Georgi Markov (who coincidentally worked for the BBC World Service at Bush House!).

The fact is that all plants, including edible ones, contain quantities of poisons. Carrots, for example, contain a nerve toxin: caratotoxin. And someone once pointed out that if cabbage had to undergo the tests that drugs are now subjected to before being pronounced fit for humans, it wouldn't pass. Lathyrism, a kind of nerve paralysis, is a disease once widespread in India, due to eating the lathyrus bean, a relation of garbanzo or chickpea. Another bean, Vicia favia, causes favism or haemolytic anaemia in sensitive individuals living around the Mediterranean Sea.

The edible nightshades (potatoes, tomatoes, capsicums, chili peppers) are especially rich sources, but cabbage, peppercorns, pulses and many other foodstuffs are not far behind. Outbreaks of food poisoning due to solanine (from potatoes), tomatine (tomatoes) and dioscorine (yams) have all been reliably observed in either humans or domestic animals. Death due to poisoning by plants is fortunately uncommon in humans; in Socrates' case (hemlock) it was deliberate murder by the state. But sub-clinical poisoning in sensitive individuals occurs all the time. This book aims to teach you facts you didn't dream of and your doctor does not suspect. Just because the majority of people can eat a food without any apparent symptoms doesn't mean everyone is genetically programmed to do so. Toxicity is a matter of degree but that is little comfort if you are one of the sensitive individuals.

Plants may also contain hormone-like substances. Oestrogen precursors are found in yams. Goitrogens are substances causing goiter (swollen neck due to thyroid enlargement). Soya bean extract includes significant amounts and goiters have been seen in human infants fed with soya milk (iodine appears to counteract this effect, so infant soya milks are fortified with iodide as a precautionary measure). Goitrogens are a common constituent of plants belonging to the Crucifer family (cabbage, turnip, swede, broccoli, cauliflower, kale, Brussels sprouts, rape and mustard seed).

Hypertensive substances are amino compounds such as serotonin and noradrenalin (norepinephrine), which constrict blood vessels and thereby elevate the blood pressure. Such substances occur in chocolate, pineapple juice, avocado, alcohol and cheese.

This is by no means an exhaustive list but sufficient to make the reader realize that there may be a problem, even if nobody has told you before. The real mystery is not so much why people are sometimes made ill by food toxins, so much as why isn't everyone made ill, all the time? (I'll give you one important answer further down.)

Poisoning may come into food indirectly. An endemic goiter seen in Tasmania is probably due to milk from cows fed on kale and turnips. A disease known as milk sickness, characterized by weakness, nausea and collapse, has occasionally reached epidemic proportions in certain parts of the USA (it probably caused the death of Abraham Lincoln's mother). The name derives from the fact that the disease is brought on by drinking milk from cows made ill with a disease known as the trembles. This was eventually tracked down to the consumption, by cattle, of a plant known as snake root (*Eupatorium rugosum*), containing the chemical tremetone. Along the same lines, a poison in lupin has been known to be transferred to human beings via goat's milk.

Plant alkaloids

One very important group of plant chemicals are the alkaloids. These are small organic molecules, usually comprising several carbon rings with side chains, one or more of the carbon atoms being replaced by a nitrogen (which confers the alkalinity). About seven to ten per cent of all plants contain alkaloids, of which several thousand are now known.

Famous alkaloids include caffeine, nicotine, quinine, strychnine, ergotamine and atropine. The less toxic ones, such as caffeine, are used for pleasant social effects or as hallucinogens (cannabis and peyote).

The action of alkaloids on the nervous system is generally to disrupt electrochemical transmission at nerve junctions (synapses), either preventing transmission (as in the case of the plant extract curare) or enhancing it inappropriately (as, for example, physostigmine).

Probably the most fascinating study of all is that of psychogenic substances in plants. Best-known are the psychedelic substances such as those in marijuana and peyote cactus; the coca plant gives rise to cocaine and the opium poppy is notorious for its forbidden juices. But there have been opium-like substances, called exorphins, found in many plants.

Exorphins are morphine-related peptides derived from partially digested grain, milk and legume proteins. Pharmacologicallythey behave, when tested on isolated tissues, very much like endorphins, hence the name (endorphins in turn, remember, are natural calming body substances named for their morphine-like properties). In people whose intestinal digestion is incomplete, exorphins are absorbed and have the effect of a small dose of an opiate drug. This may be one of the main reasons that some people find food very soporific and tend to fall asleep after a heavy meal.

Finally, think of the caffeine family (known as methylxanthines). It is commonly overlooked that caffeine and theobromine (which occur in tea, coffee and chocolate) are toxic substances. Taken in sufficient quantities they can cause cerebral edema (so-called 'water on the brain'), convulsions and even death, though no one has ever been able to establish tissue damage caused by chronic ingestion at normal levels. However I know from my own work that methylxanthines are a potent cause of chronic mastitis in women, sometimes called fibrocystic disease of the breasts – sore "lumpy" breasts. This complaint gives rise to a great deal of anxiety and sometimes leads to complications. The cure is very simple and satisfying: cut the coffee and chocolate!

Let me just conclude here by saying that the animal kingdom does not escape this wide sweep of food toxins: consider the puffer fish, or fugu. The tetrodotoxin from its liver is so potent that a tiny trace contaminating a knife can kill a man. In Japan, where eating fugu is a macho-bravura cult, chefs must be specially licensed and trained to handle this delicacy safely. Nevertheless, there have been many unfortunate deaths due to this cause.

3

The Myths of Nutritional Medicine

I t is no big secret that eating right keeps you healthy. Hundreds of thousands of papers are published every year, describing scientific studies which have looked at some aspect of this issue and come to the same inevitable conclusion. The only people who don't seem to have heard the good news are members of the medical profession! I'm not speaking disparagingly of individual doctors – many of my colleagues are very switched on to nutrition and diet – but it is a sad truth that the vast majority of practicing physicians and surgeons have either never heard of the benefits of good nutrition, or have disregarded it or have remained so pathetically ignorant of what is required that they neither teach nor apply the principles of good diet to their suffering patients.

A really cynical critic would argue that maybe the doctors don't want their patients restored to health and happiness; that they only want dollars for treating conditions that could be resolved naturally. That may be too harsh. I think the trouble is that doctors never get past Nutrition 101 in med school. Instead of becoming competent with this vital tool, they are taught only falsehoods and half-truths.

Doctors have it drummed into them that:

- Fats are bad for us, whereas in fact certain fats are essential to survival and form part of our all-important cell membranes. Gosh, even our brains are forty percent fat; how would we even think without good clean fats? Low fat diets I see handed out by doctors are destructive to health because some of our vitamins can only be absorbed in the presence of fats (A, E and D). These vitamins in turn enhance the absorption of essential minerals.

- Carbohydrates are desirable and build health; in fact they contribute virtually nothing, other than obesity and insulin problems. White flour and starch have no nutrient qualities; over 90% of B vitamins are removed and only a small fraction of that added back in "vitamin enriched" flours. Even so-called complex carbohydrates, the natural ones, are bad in excess. Consider that farmers, with an eye to profits, fatten up their livestock by feeding them large quantities of carbohydrate.

- Only trace doses of vitamins or minerals are necessary for health. The truth is these are merely the levels needed to prevent us dying horribly of scurvy, beri-beri and the like. The so-called recommended dietary allowances (RDAs) bear no relation to the quantities needed for optimum health and do not take into account basic scientific variables, such as the fact that we are all biologically different, we need a higher intake under different conditions, notably disease and stress, or that we may not even be absorbing our nutrients properly!

- Doses of vitamins even slightly above daily allowance levels *may* be dangerous. This is especially ironic when doctors tend to cling to the biochemical nonsense that some is good, so more is better (drug dosages). In fact pet food contains doses many times above the supposed safe levels for humans: if you allow for the body weight of smaller mammals, the levels recommended for a healthy beast are hundreds of times greater than those for humans!

- A "balanced diet" will give you all the essential nutrients you need. A balance of what exactly? Junk? Most foods on the supermarket shelf are vitiated make-overs of what Nature has supplied and thus severely depleted of essential nutrients. Take zinc as an example: this vital mineral helps build our tissues and maintain immunity. But modern farming methods leave even the soil deficient in zinc. It cannot be taken up by crops and the livestock that feeds on the land; thus the whole food chain is zinc deficient in most areas. It is not possible to obtain adequate doses of this nutrient from your diet, however varied!

- Food allergy and intolerance is very rare. Officially, figures still claim that food allergy affects only between 1% and 7% of the population. This is misleading, and such statistics concern only extremely violent food reactions that we call "immediate hypersensitivity" and which sometimes leads to anaphylaxis and death. But the kind of food allergy you are going to read about in this book is different. It is subtler and often remains in disguise. The official position is therefore false euphoria, and until doctors are taught to diagnose the problem properly, this sort of underestimation of the problem will continue.

The list could go on and on. This does not even take into account that most physicians have never even heard of the problem of genetic variations leading to individual unique food incompatibilities. I'm sure you've got the point. Nonsense at this level is passed 'round and 'round and repeated so often that it has become accepted as "scientific" and therefore true.

Nor are doctors the only ones who are guilty of ignorance and disinformation. The major secrets I will reveal to you in this book are largely unknown or disregarded by other health workers too, each with their own axe to grind. There are an astonishing number of allergy "experts" out there, offering advice and treatment, who have never been through med school, and many of them, from what I read, have not even studied basic physiology.

You need to be informed in order to be protected. In any case, this is a field where you really can do most of the investigations yourself, with a little care and patience and by following closely the "game rules" I will explain. That's right: I often liken this to a game of allergy and intolerance – there are rules which you need to know, otherwise you cannot win. But they are not complicated or mysterious rules, just little known, except to a few. We can dispose of many health problems, but always remember this: if you have an allergy tendency or a genetic food incompatibility, it won't go away. You need to be *food wise* all your life.

Four big secrets to healthy eating

I'm going to let you in on the two biggest secrets to healthy eating that I know. I'm doing it now, rather than tease, so that you can begin to re-align everything you know or have read, or think you know, with what follows in this book, while bearing these important revolutionary facts in mind.

Ultimate Diet Principle 1.

Eating what you shouldn't does far more harm than not eating what you should. This is the opposite of parental nagging, which says things like "Eat your greens," and "You need the calcium in milk for strong bones and teeth." Everyone has certain foods which react un-typically; which stress up their metabolism and are poorly tolerated. No matter how important the food, or "essential" it is for your well being, if you eat such a toxic food you will be ill.

Similarly, if you follow the dietary recommendations of someone who has not heard of food allergy or genetic food incompatibility, you may find yourself feeling worse. Whereas some foods are commoner allergies than others, I have patients allergic or intolerant to every single so-called healthy food you could name: lettuce, bananas, fish, apples, tomatoes, whole wheat, herbal teas and all the rest of the healthy foods that are supposed to be good for you. I have yet to see a popular diet book that even acknowledges this crucial health factor, let alone makes allowance for it.

That's why this book is important: it fills a vital gap in knowledge.

The exact mechanism of incompatibility is not important to this key understanding. I am not confining my remarks to food allergies, intolerance or any other mechanism. Nor is it necessary, for the success of this plan, that you identify why you do not tolerate the food. The important step is to identify such stressor foods and remove them from your diet. You will benefit immediately from increased well being, zest and health. Many chronic symptoms you may have become accustomed to and consider almost "normal" will disappear.

Ultimate Diet Principle 2.

These toxic or incompatible foods are different for everyone. Thus there can be no one-size-fits-all diet. Diets do not really work by giving you "good" foods, but by taking you off the bad foods.

Those diets that succeed in any degree at all really do so because of Principle 1, often inadvertently and without anyone being aware of the real reason. By following a suggested eating plan, the individual must avoid certain foods and the real benefit comes from this exclusion principle. The credit for the recovery is given to the new diet craze and the correct scientific explanation, which I am giving you here in this book, remains obscure.

For example: you may have heard of the "food combining" approach to diet. A lot of elaborate theory is put forward as a justification for the ritual of separating morning, midday and evening – your body is supposed to be unable to digest proteins and carbohydrates at the same time, some foods are acid and some are alkaline and other such fake science. These claims are simply not true. The body is geared to digest fats, carbohydrates and proteins, sequentially, in different segments of the alimentary tract.

But what I observe is that individuals on the food combining program simply avoid or drastically reduce their intake of certain foods.

For example the breakfast is supposed to be fruit. That means no toast and no cereals (and therefore very probably little or no milk). Those two simple changes are enough to make the majority of the population feel healthier, because grains, especially wheat and dairy products are the two most common incompatible foods. I estimate that over 80% of the population are intolerant to one or the other, or both. That means a great many people are going to feel better while on the food combining diet; in other words, excluding foods. We don't need any hokey food science to explain that.

From what you have just read there follow two more very important diet principles that you need to understand and remember:

Ultimate Diet Principle 3.

All published set diets make a percentage of people worse because they are forced to eat *more* of their toxic foods. You can take it as a further "rule" that you just don't get to hear of these failures! The author of the latest best-selling diet just does not know or does not care about the failures. In true medico-style it is the patient who is blamed: the unlucky individual is shrugged off as "atypical" or just plain difficult.

The vast majority of patients who do feel unwell, naturally, never bother to report to the author of the diet what has happened. They maybe blame themselves, feel worse and just quit the diet with a sigh, hoping the next plan might be the one for them.

So for all the hype and success stories you hear, whatever the diet, just remember the luckless individuals who got *worse*!

Ultimate Diet Principle 4.

There is only one diet that is right for you and you must figure it out for yourself.

You need to know which are your *personal* toxic foods and avoid those, possibly for life, though there are exceptions to this, as we shall see. How to work out this crucial knowledge is one of the most important steps you will ever take in regard to your health. The major part of this book is devoted to helping you in this quest for safe, harmonious and user-friendly eating.

The only way to find out for sure what's happening with you is to test it yourself, using the best available test instrument we have – your own body. *Diet Wise* is much more than just an eating plan: I will show you the principles involved, what steps to take and how to interpret the results reliably, so that you can acquire vital knowledge you will need to enjoy a long and healthy life.

This is the ultimate workable plan because it is a custom-fit!

Let's get started with some explanatory theory. In the coming chapters I'll tell you all you need to know in order to succeed, and probably even more than you need. These ideas are not theoretical but intensely practical, the techniques I myself used every day in my office for over three decades; and everything you will read here has been tried and tested thousands of times. It is a *working* system, and as such it has a great deal to commend it.

4

Cases, Cases, Cases

To give you some idea of what can be achieved, here are some case histories from my clinical notebooks. These are not even the most sensational recoveries I know of. The ones included here are typical of a wide variety of conditions and are chosen because they show ordinary people with ordinary, though in some cases severe, diseases – the kind you might be suffering from. These are not medical reports of the kind that I would supply to a fellow medical practitioner, just plain stories, told in everyday English that illustrate the point. The scientific and technical basis of these recoveries are fully covered later in the book. Each case was put through the *diet wise* plan and the results are summarized. Long before the final chapter you should be able to achieve the same success for yourself. The trick is to work out what your own *personal ideal diet* is.

Case no. 1: Severe arthritis

Mac was a friendly 50-year-old Scot, lively, intelligent and well educated – everything the emigré from north of the border of Britain is traditionally noted for. He was hard-working and successful too, one of the army of quiet businessmen of the type who once helped Britain build and maintain her empire across the globe. At the peak of his career he was senior executive in a Far Eastern company, traveling the world and enjoying the respect of colleagues from Manchester to Tokyo. He had earned his status and was entitled to be proud of it.

Then arthritis struck. At first it was no more than an uncomfortable periodic ache, but unfortunately it soon progressed and began to worsen with relentless speed. Within a few years he was a very sick man and his way of life had become very restricted. The pain was severe, but the main enemy was stiffness: some days it would take him one-and-a half hours to get out of bed and get moving sufficiently to leave the house or hotel. Although he tried to conceal his difficulty, it soon became obvious to his workfellows. Instead of enjoying his work as he always had, he suddenly found in it only embarrassment and physical discomfort.

Things drifted for a while. Various doctors treated him, but this amounted to no more than painkillers, which did little to help and made no impact on the progress of the disease. Inevitably, it became impossible for him to do his job, energy consuming and demanding as it was. The final straw came in Japan – a heart attack which was followed by angina: pain due to cardiac under-perfusion brought on by exercise. Mac was pensioned off, so to speak, on health grounds and sent home to this country. There he was given work that was much easier, but it was very unfulfilling for someone like him. He felt as if he had been relegated to the back row, and it cast a long, deep shadow on all his achievements and his career as a whole.

By the time he came to my clinic he was an unhappy and frustrated man. His body was causing him great anguish, and his mind had begun to lose the razor-sharp edge to which he had always been accustomed. His speech was broken up by embarrassingly long pauses while he tried to resume his train of thought. It is particularly sad when a condition of this sort brings down the "big" ones: men and women of great zest and skill, the "doers" in life that most of us envy. They take it very hard. And to add to his gloom, he had been told by every doctor he had spoken to that his debility was permanent and "incurable"; they said he would have to "live with it," (a favorite phrase, and an unbearably depressing one).

From the first I suspected food allergies. High-fliers are often high-livers, and a study of his diet showed this to be the case. I explained to him the *diet wise* plan (I don't call it that with patients; the correct name is elimination and challenge dieting) and he started on it. To his immense delight, within ten days he noticed an improvement. The pain and swelling in his joints began to subside. He started waking with a clear head and a body that responded within minutes instead of hours. He wasn't of an age to leap out of bed, but in contrast to the way he had been that was how it felt to him. Each day, especially the mornings, again became something to look forward to instead of to dread. On his second visit he looked and felt a new man.

We then set about finding out which foods had been causing the trouble. I allowed him to slowly, one at a time and over a few weeks, reintroduce the foods he had been avoiding. Those which caused a recurrence of his symptoms he was instructed to steer clear of. If there was no reaction, that food was considered safe and allowed to remain in his diet.

In this way we discovered he was allergic to a number of foods, but in particular wheat (the worst), chicken and orange. Providing he avoids them he remains happy and reasonably well. It isn't a complete recovery, but enough to allow him to do as he wishes, namely work, travel to the Far East several times a year and generally pick up life where he had left off. As an added bonus, his angina has disappeared completely: he is off all drugs and is capable of carrying out normal physical activities, even a full round of golf, without pain.

Yet if he eats wheat, especially bread, his symptoms return with a vengeance – so much so that he no longer tries to test it and avoids it completely, even in gravy thickening. As he sees it, it simply isn't worth the trouble and pain; it is far easier to eat differently as outlined in this book. A miracle? He thinks so, and I must admit that even after all this time I haven't lost my sense of wonder when someone gets well like that.

Case no. 2: Mysterious swellings

Mrs. G was a 47-year-old married social worker. Apart from being a little highly strung, she had enjoyed good health for most of her adult life. She had raised three fine children and was approaching the time of life when she and her husband would be entitled to start looking forward to enjoying the fruits of their labors.

The dream of a comfortable middle age was, however, rudely shattered by sudden ill health: not cancer, high blood pressure, a coronary or any of the well-known sinister and dangerous conditions, yet to her it was frightening and debilitating and it had a hardly less damaging effect on her well being than possible more serious complaints might have done. About four years before she came to see me, sudden mysterious swellings had started to develop. These were not continually present but came in attacks that occurred every few weeks right out of the blue.

There was no pattern to it: there might be several occurrences in a month, or alternatively none for many weeks. Her face was most prominently affected, and when the condition was severe her eyes would close up completely. Sometimes the throat was involved and the swelling would press on the windpipe, making breathing difficult; she would then be forced to tilt her head back in order to get air in and out of her lungs. Naturally, these episodes were quite terrifying. A doctor would be rushed to her for emergency treatment, but there was always the haunting fear that she might suffocate before help arrived.

It was no ordinary puffiness but a huge increase in size: her head would feel almost too heavy to lift because of the great weight of fluid. She looked like a gargoyle, grotesque and unnatural, so much so that her friends could hardly recognize her. Of course, she was quite unable to work for fear of scaring her clients. The protuberances would disappear as mysteriously as they had come, only to return at some point later. Doctors were unable to diagnose the reason or to help. It was no use staying permanently on drugs when there was no way of knowing when the condition would strike next. The attacks were getting to be more frequent, and by the time we met she was depressed and desperate.

My first question was "When did it start?" She remembered the occasion clearly. It was in a traffic jam, she had been driving her car and had, like most of the other drivers, become steadily more frustrated and overwrought mentally. The fumes had been choking, and the heat (it was a summer's day) had made her feel faint and weary. When the traffic eventually got on the move again she had found herself in tears: perhaps it was due to stress, or to the fact that her eyes felt red and itchy – she wasn't sure. But by the time she got home and looked in the mirror the truth was obvious: some strange and frightening reaction had caused her face to puff up and her eyes to turn bloodshot and sore. After that the problem recurred with increasing frequency. It would be tempting to assume an allergy to traffic fumes, but it is worth noting that she was exposed on a very large number of occasions to equally high concentrations and had no reaction. Furthermore, she would sometimes get this swelling without even going out of doors. Inconsistencies like this are fully explained in this book.

Having drawn up a full history of her case, I found plenty of supportive symptoms, such as aching muscles, a general slowing down, insomnia and flu-like attacks (that were not flu), to suggest allergy, including food allergy, as the cause of the trouble. So we discussed the plan given in this book and she decided to give it a try.

To cut the rest of the story short, the treatment was a complete success. She carried out tests on herself using the procedure outlined in a later chapter and found it was best to avoid certain foods: *wheat, corn, chicken,* cheese, egg, milk and coffee (the items in italics were the worst offenders). Since then there has been no recurrence of her condition; not only that, but she feels fitter and healthier than she can remember being in years. I fully expected to have to delve into chemical sensitivities, but this turned out to be unnecessary. Not that this proves she is not intolerant of chemicals; simply that, with her diet under control, she can cope with these as well as the rest of us can.

I have encountered this theme time and time again and can formulate it as a simple rule of management: deal with dietary intolerance first and many other conditions simply recover, as the overload effect disappears.

Case no. 3: Behavioral problems

The next case is that of a schoolboy which is so like the story of hundreds and thousands of others that I think it a great shame that all teachers, as well as parents, are unaware of the importance of diet in influencing behavior. Luckily this tale has a happy ending, but so many do not: often delinquency, even crime, follows in the wake of poor eating, and the helpless teachers and mystified parents never suspect the real reason. Such a pity, when the cure is so easy, as this book shows.

I have allowed the lad's mother to tell the story in the form of a letter to me:

Dear Dr. Scott-Mumby,

It's marvelous to be able to write and tell you what a complete success your dietary program has been with our son Alan. As you know, we had some awful problems, but now, thanks to you, he is the lovely boy he promised to be as a toddler. Let me go back to the beginning.

Alan as a little baby was always so happy and a delight to be with. In fact we had no inkling of what was to follow. It wasn't until he reached the age of about three, when he started to go to preschool, that things began to go wrong.

We were told that he behaved rather aggressively towards the other children and that he was demanding and seemed to want the attention of the group leader all the time. We were surprised, because this was so untypical. We talked it over and assumed it was just a phase he was going through and that he needed time to adjust. But in fact it got worse.

Then we suspected that he had communication problems. Although quite bright and certainly not backward for his age, his speech was virtually non-existent. We decided this should be tackled vigorously and, after much cajoling, we managed to get professional help from a succession of speech therapists. This paid off in the sense that his speech is now almost perfect, unlike that of many of his peers. But his behavior, unfortunately, did not improve.

When he started school we became very worried about his attitude to everything and everybody; his moods seemed to swing from being loving and caring to becoming an uncooperative and introverted little "monkey" [sic].

Over the next couple of years things got worse and worse. Although we knew for certain that he was bright, he was consistently underachieving in his studies and we were told he was a disruptive influence on the rest of the class. He was always in trouble, he would "forget" to bring home his homework, and we would get frequent disturbing phone calls from the headmistress telling us what a problem he was. She had tried many times to admonish or discipline him, but nothing she – or we – said seemed to have any effect.

It wasn't only school that was affected: it began to be noticeable he was being invited out less and less and his friends became fewer. One day we were told by a helpful parent that it was because his moods swung so violently from happy to surly, aggressive and back. It was so unpredictable that it was most disconcerting for others.

Then he began to complain of tummy ache in the mornings. At first we thought this was just a ruse to get out of going to school, but he had it during the holidays also. Headaches began to follow, and we finally started to take him seriously when he told us he was getting pains in his joints, mainly the legs. The doctor said it was nothing to worry about, just "growing pains," but that didn't seem right to us.

Meanwhile his behavior was worse than ever. We tried coaxing, smacking, cuddling and penalties over the years, but nothing had any effect. He would do all sorts of strange, destructive things, such as ripping pajamas, tearing books, smashing up, etc., and when we asked him why he did it he would break down and cry. He had no idea why he was doing it – he certainly didn't want to behave like that and it was pitiful to watch the conflict going on inside him. We felt so helpless.

Then one day we heard of you and your clinic. We thought anything was worth a try. Since then we have never looked back. He has reverted to being a normal, sociable young boy, we are free of the tension and worry, and he is so happy and calm it is a pleasure to watch him.

We are not pretending that sticking to the diet has been easy. It is very restrictive for someone his age. But we have explained to Alan that it isn't forever, maybe just eighteen months or two years. So long as he keeps to it, all is well.

We have begun to reintroduce certain foods, albeit gradually, to his diet. The ones he cannot tolerate are withdrawn again. This way we have a very clear idea of what foods affect him. It seems doubtful if he will ever be able to take eggs in any great amount. When he eats anything with egg in he immediately gets a headache and pains in his chest, stomach and joints. It's a pity we keep our own hens!

We have had one or two ups and downs. A few weeks ago Alan crept into the kitchen while we were sleeping and demolished half a cake and some cookies. The following day he was dreadful. All his antisocial mannerisms returned. At first we had no idea why but when we found the empty cake tin we were naturally angry. But we should not have been; he was very remorseful and knew he had been silly. I suppose it was a valuable lesson.

His teachers and tutor are amazed at the transformation. His schoolwork has improved dramatically. He brings home extra work by choice, his concentration span is far longer, and in class he is cheerful and cooperative.

The fraught atmosphere in the home has gone. He is often invited out for tea now and several mothers have approached me and told me what a delight he now is to have in their homes. It's bliss! We still have to shake ourselves to believe that it's true and just how lucky we were to find your clinic. If we hadn't, I'm sure he would have been under the care of a child or educational psychologist, and what would have become of our loved son by now is open to question.

The ironic thing is, before we met you I had always assumed we were having an extremely balanced diet; I think I told you I am a caterer and dietician by profession. I was wrong. All that has changed now. I understand about food allergies and, as a family, our eating habits have changed dramatically. We all look and feel much healthier!

Once again, thank you.
Mrs. B

Case no. 4: Eczema

This case concerns Mr. Exley, a 41-year-old man with severe eczema, an unpleasant peeling, weeping and cracking condition of the skin. His face was like a mask, and the eczema extended all over his body, worse in some parts than others. He was an architect, and meeting clients caused him intense embarrassment, so much so that he felt like apologizing for himself. At its worst the rash was so bad that he had to be wrapped in bandages soaked in cold water to overcome the intense irritation. It had first started about four years before he came to me, and within the first twelve months he had been in trouble: he had then needed to be kept in the hospital for three weeks on steroid medication.

These drugs *appear* wonderful at producing a rapid cure, but there is always a sting in the tail: once you start them you can't easily stop them, or the condition will flare up again. You see, they *never* cure, only mask symptoms. That's exactly what happened to Mr. Exley. Three weeks after he was sent home, the rash was worse than ever. He did not succeed in abandoning the steroid creams altogether, but managed to cope with his condition, very wretchedly, for over three more years.

Finally, in desperation, he came to see if I could help. In his case there were few corroborating symptoms to suggest the cause of the rash, but I regard eczema as *always* being an ecological-based disease. If anyone needs convincing, take note of the important clue he gave me: each summer when he goes for a long holiday in the sun it clears up completely. (Rest and sunshine is not the reason, as you will read in a later chapter, but a change of diet). This proved that, intrinsically, there was nothing wrong with him or his body – *not a thing*.

This leads to a second Scott-Mumby rule I developed over the years. As I have always said to patients: *if you can be well on one day, you can be well every day*! Think about it.

All we had to do was locate what substances were causing such unpleasant skin reactions. I thought it highly probable that food was to blame, and I told him so. I explained the plan to him and assured him that though it was tough at first it represented his best road forward. He considered he had nothing to lose by trying and so agreed. He started the diet stage immediately.

This time there was no dramatic improvement on the elimination step. During the withdrawal phase (which you will read about) his skin at times hung off like shreds of tattered wallpaper; but after three weeks, although his skin was somewhat better, I knew we hadn't succeeded fully. Either he was not allergic to the omitted foods or something he was being allowed to continue in his diet did not agree with him. Yet it would have been a terrible mistake to assume he was not reacting to any of the banned foods; in fact, when we tested them several caused a flare-up, namely wheat, egg (very bad), tomato and milk.

We next went on to inquire into several foods we regard as *relatively* safe. (The emphasized word is important because there is no such thing as an absolutely safe food: I have patients who have been made ill by every substance you can name, including such innocent-sounding ones as carrot, lettuce and water.)

In Mr. Exley's case we came up trumps with pork and lamb. For both of these he followed the outlined test procedure given in this plan, and there was no mistaking the result: it meant several days of feeling unwell with a raw, itchy skin. Avoiding those also, he began to make rapid progress, and within weeks his skin looked clear and healthy except for small patches on his lower legs. Since none of his clients see this part of him it causes no embarrassment or difficulty, and naturally he is very pleased.

Case no. 5: Bowel disorder

The next patient is Maria, an attractive 24-year-old Londoner of Cypriot extraction. She came to see me with abdominal distress, flatulence, bloating and variability of bowel function. Sometimes she would be constipated for days on end; at others she had diarrhea so severely that she would be caught out and have to run immediately to the nearest toilet. The complaint had troubled her for as long as she could remember; furthermore, her father, *his* father, an aunt and a young cousin were affected in exactly the same way.

Almost continual stomach pains were bad enough, but what troubled her most was the flatulence. She had a job that meant a lot to her: working for a celebrity tour promotion agency. It meant she had frequent opportunities to accompany artists and stars for up to a day, taking them for meals and showing them around the capital. But so often had she declined these wonderful assignments (using fabricated excuses about "important appointments") that her employers had assumed she was not interested and ceased to ask her. Instead she was left with mundane office chores, and even then things were sometimes difficult; she had to suddenly excuse herself from a meeting to break wind in the corridor outside.

Her relationships with the opposite sex were spoilt because she was embarrassed about her condition. She had a fixation that she smelt offensive, and one boyfriend, perhaps trying to be helpful, had dropped hints about this, indicating that it was not all "in her mind." When the symptoms were particularly bad she preferred to stay at home rather than mix with others, making up feeble excuses. Few men were prepared to put up with her apparent indifference and to persist. Her current boyfriend was a little more understanding, but she refused to see him very often and could not bring herself to tell him why. Naturally, he was puzzled and thought her a strange girl.

Apart from the bowel disorder Maria also occasionally suffered from panic attacks, when everything seemed to press in on her. At these times she would experience the fright of impending doom and feel certain she was about to die. However, her overriding emotion was not anxiety but deep despair and gloom; she frequently felt so depressed that suicide seemed the only answer, she confided in me.

Fortunately she had never tried it, otherwise she would have ended up in the hands of some psychiatrist and the outcome might not have been so happy. She had been admitted to the hospital twice for investigations, but all tests had proved negative. The final diagnosis (which is no diagnosis at all) was a "lazy colon," and she was prescribed drugs, which failed to help. Disillusioned and cynical, she had long since given up seeing her family doctor.

I inquired into her diet with my routine inventory (see Chapter 10), and she told me she was eating largely whole foods, including plenty of fruit and vegetables, both fresh and simply cooked. She ate very few canned and packaged meals and no junk food, except on birthdays and at the seaside: on the surface of it, not a very high-risk diet. But then I knew that *any* food was a *potential* allergen.

I explained to Maria that since her digestive tract appeared to bear the brunt of symptoms, food allergy or intolerance was very probable. She liked the sound of the approach used in the *diet wise* plan and decided to give it a try.

Within ten days she had made startling progress: the flatulence had ceased completely, her abdominal pains had dropped to a tenth of their former level, and she felt *wonderful*. Her stomach was now flat instead of bloated. Energy and confidence radiated from her. She told me confidentially that her libido was on the increase. The black moods had lifted, and she now considered herself equal to any social or work pressure that might come her way.

From then on she never looked back. Apart from occasions when she deliberately tested a food and experienced a reaction, her symptoms have not returned. Subsequently we found she was allergic to cabbage, cauliflower, turnip (all members of the mustard family), potato, lamb, pork, wheat, egg and tomato. She had been eating one or another of these foods every day yet had never suspected them to be the trouble: none had ever caused an obvious symptom that had aroused her suspicions. Nevertheless, within a few days on this plan, carrying out the correct procedure as outlined by me, she was able to demonstrate a pronounced reaction to each of the above foods. Incidentally, egg seemed to be the cause of most of the flatulence: within minutes of the test dose she was breaking offensive wind – long before any egg could possibly have reached the lower bowel.

Her work is now her greatest pleasure, and she accepts the hostess assignments without hesitation, rubbing shoulders with VIPs and celebrities, at ease and, by all accounts, popular – after all, she knows London better than most native Britons do.

Case no. 6: Schizophrenia

A young man I shall call Tony came to my clinic, and I think it would be no exaggeration to state that his life was in ruins due to unsuspected food allergies. His story has all the human drama you could wish for outside the fantasy annals of Dr. Kildare. He came from a good home, had enjoyed normal health as a child, did well at school and at eleven-plus age there had been no clouds on his life's horizon. His secondary education had started off well: he had shown himself to be very bright, and his teachers had expected him to be very successful in the public examinations when he was sixteen.

Then a double tragedy struck: his grandfather, to whom he was very close, died suddenly, and within a very short interval a close friend committed suicide. People die all the time, of course, with varying degrees of impact on those they leave behind; but for an adolescent boy facing the stress of preparation for major examinations it proved rather a lot to cope with. Tony's mood changed, and he began to suffer long bouts of gloom. At times he became so indolent with despondency that it quite worried his parents. They sought medical advice, with the result that at the incredibly early age of fourteen he was put on antidepressant drugs. These are a disaster at any age, in my opinion, but to prescribe them for a newly forming adult personality was an unforgivable blunder.

Despite it all Tony struggled on at school, and few people knew his troubles. There was therefore much consternation and surprise when he failed badly in his exams. Doubtless being dosed up on psychotropic (mind-altering) drugs had a lot to do with this. He was allowed to stay on nevertheless, but in the sixth form his behavior progressively deteriorated: his bouts of depression caused him to become truculent, moody and unreasonable. Finally, even his friends were alienated. At this stage he was diagnosed as a case of schizophrenia.

Sadly, he failed his next level examinations and his promising academic career came to an end. He had been offered a university place on the strength of his known abilities, but was unable to go. Even a most understanding faculty could not permit a student to matriculate without justifiable exam results; it simply would not be fair to other students competing for a place.

So Tony ended up working in a library. It was work that held no interest for him and failed to challenge his intellect. There were no prospects that stimulated him, and it was, in every sense, a dead-end job: in other words, in all normal social terms he was a failure, and knew it, which only served to enhance his general mood of depression. Life was a drudge that could only be borne by taking frequent large doses of drugs, and by this time he was having one of these by injection – all this, remember, before he was twenty. What could possibly have gone wrong to snuff out such a promising bright spark?

Actually, there were many clues for the person who knew what to look for: while he was in the hospital a skin rash was noticed which passed without comment; he suffered from headaches, palpitations and sudden tiredness after eating; his mood was particularly bad first thing in the morning and breakfast helped him feel better; also, he was occasionally gripped by eating binges. These and other signs made it very obvious to me that Tony had food allergies.

He was put on the diet given in Chapter 11 and followed the plan outlined in this book. Within days he began to improve, and within a fortnight an astonishing change had taken place. He described it as being like waking up after years of sleep. His mind cleared as if a fog had lifted, and for the first time in years he was able to look towards the future and feel it was something friendly instead of hostile; for him it was a time of new horizons. He began to reduce the amount of drugs he took. He was a new human being, cheerful and sociable. The nightmare which had begun as a bereavement was finally at an end.

Subsequent tests showed him to be allergic to a wide variety of the foods he had been eating regularly. The worst offenders were cane sugar, milk, cheese, apple, chocolate and tomato, while others included chicken, potato, wheat, egg, yeast and rice – hardly surprising, therefore, that he was ill! Since then he has made plans to restart his studies: there is no question that both his ability to concentrate and the right motivation have returned.

5

Definition Time

L et's start with a few terms: you can't expect to understand a new topic unless you become familiar with the use of its special words or jargon.

We need to establish two specific phenomena: food allergy proper and food intolerance caused by genetic factors and specific metabolic incompatibilities to foods.

To begin with, what do we mean by *allergy?* It is actually not a very straightforward term, though it is used a lot. The word was first coined in 1906 by an Austrian physician, Von Pirquet, so obviously he had the right to say what he meant by it. He specified it as 'an acquired, specific, altered capacity to react to physical substances on the part of the body.'

Note the word *acquired:* it means you do not inherit the sensitivity. This is not like the toxic venom of a snake, where the first dose is just as harmful as later doses.

According to our understanding of the allergy mechanism, you need to be exposed to the substance before you develop a reaction to it. This exposure may be as slight as one prior contact, yet it must take place. It is confusing, perhaps, that many infants are born with allergies, but that does not violate this stipulation. The fact is that babies in the womb are exposed to a great many potentially allergenic substances via the mother's diet and bloodstream. This is how we think they acquire the sensitivity.

The term *specific* means that the reaction associated with a particular substance is quite unique, even though the results may not be. Thus tomato may make you ill, and so may house dust, but the reacting mechanism in each case is not the same, though the symptom that is caused may well be.

Altered is really a way of saying that it is peculiar to the individual in question, not something that the rest of us are troubled by. This is important, for otherwise we fail to distinguish the special problems of allergy from those of straightforward poisoning. Thus cyanide or muscarine (from the toadstool *Aminita muscaria)* would make everyone ill – these are poisons. But some individuals are made ill by simple substances such as milk, coffee and egg, and this is not normal. These foods cause no trouble for the majority of the population, and so, for some people, this is an *altered* (abnormal) reaction.

There is, however, a certain amount of overlap between allergy and poisoning effects: for example, house gas makes us all ill in sufficient concentration, but there are an unlucky few who react even to the tiniest traces of it, traces so small that the concentration will not register on instruments from the gas supply board. Are they simply being poisoned at an earlier stage, or is this a special *altered* reaction on their part that we may call an allergy? Often it is difficult to decide. But fortunately we do not need to make up our minds between the two phenomena: in the end, if the patient feels better for avoiding that particular substance, *that* is what counts.

Doctors cling to the narrow dismissive view

Some doctors went on to extend Von Pirquet's work and discovered that *some* allergy reactions were mediated by antibodies (special chemicals provoked by the encounter) and certain lymphocytes, a type of white blood cell – very interesting. Next this was followed by an insistence that *only* those reactions that involved demonstrable antibodies and/or lymphocytes could be called allergies. This is an extraordinarily narrow and arrogant viewpoint. Other reactions are then dismissed as – what? *"All in the mind"* is a common label. It isn't very scientific to dismiss phenomena for which we have no explanation as "imaginary," and it is especially hurtful to the poor patient, who has not only to bear this insulting jibe but also to continue to suffer the illness because no one will take it seriously.

I have even heard doctors insist that food and chemicals *could not possibly* make people unwell, simply because antibodies cannot be shown. They stick to this idiotic viewpoint despite the existence of hundreds of thousands of documented recoveries. Because they believe the patients to be neurotic or "imagining" their symptoms, their usual explanation for all these astonishing recoveries is that the patient responds because "someone is taking an interest" in his or her case. (Don't laugh – I have heard this on many occasions.) These gentlemen, and quite a few ladies, are not troubled by mere facts, only by the entrenchment of obscure pet theories.

Since I first wrote this cry of disbelief (1984) it has now become accepted that small chemical molecules can contribute, even to the "classical" allergy response: so-called *haptens*. Furthermore, chemical pollution, such as traffic fumes, has been admitted as a trigger for symptoms in sensitive individuals. The acceptance of food allergy in recent years has moved outside the acute antigen-antibody model, known as Type I hypersensitivity, and now includes recognition of serum antigen-antibody complexes, giving rise to widespread organ sickness, as I and other pioneers have been writing about for decades.

It often comes as a shock to patients to realize that doctors rarely seem excited and enthusiastic about each new breakthrough in healing. Medicine has a particularly bad history in this respect: almost every new advance has had to be fought for in the teeth of severe opposition. There seems to be a peculiar, almost sinister, aspect to the medical profession that makes it resistant to new ideas. Unfortunately, of course, this works to the detriment of patients, who trustingly believe their own physician to be abreast of new developments without realizing that he or she may be actively opposed to an idea *without ever having tried it out personally.*

Practical experience validates food allergies

One of the reasons the food allergy and genetic food intolerance phenomenon was opposed for so many years was that tests for it are unreliable. Most physicians, as you know, like lab work. They even give it more respect than the patient's own story: "We have your lab work and there is nothing wrong with you," is a common way of dismissing a suffering patient who apparently cannot be helped. It is a mystery to me why colleagues never seem to ask themselves the obvious question: *Is there anything wrong with the lab reports? Are we missing something here?*

Most of them would never dream of testing for food allergies and have never even heard of gene testing to establish food incompatibilities, so it is not surprising they miss the problem and tell the patient "It's all in your head." Unfortunately, even the conscientious physician is likely to be misled by current methods of detecting food allergies. The old-fashioned scratch of prick tests hardly ever show reactions, even when the patient reports being violently ill after eating the food. Newer tests for genetic profiles remain very expensive and are simply not used routinely.

So what do we do?

It's simple really. We rely on practical strategies. With or without supportive blood work or metabolic profiling, if the patient recovers after avoiding a food, that means it is highly likely to be a problem, whether it is allergy, intolerance or the toxic overload effect described in Chapter 8. Even the layman easily understands the concept of "something to avoid," which is pretty well the broadest interpretation of allergy or intolerance I use here in this book. The mechanism isn't important; recognition and avoidance is.

We can use a practical, *working* definition of an allergy, whether to a food or any other substance. A substance is considered to be an allergen if:

- firstly, the patient feels better on avoiding it;
- secondly, he or she becomes ill again on re-exposure to it;
- and thirdly, no other obvious cause for the symptoms can be shown.

The 'eight nails in the shoe' trap

The first two criteria must be capable of being repeated on more than one occasion. Yet there are certain catches to this that must be understood, or the unwary or casual observer will be tripped up. For example, the patient may not feel better merely by virtue of avoiding one allergy substance. If several others are also causing trouble, why should that person feel well, unless he or she avoids them also?

This is what Dr. Doris Rapp, one of the great American ladies of medicine, refers to as the "eight nails in the shoe" trap. If you have eight nails sticking up in your shoe, you will surely limp. If you draw four or even six of these, it may be no use – you still limp because of the remainder. You need to get rid of all eight for a proper recovery.

Metaphorically speaking, it is the same with allergies and intolerance. Numerous patients have come to me and explained that they had tried giving up, say, milk for a few weeks and felt no better; therefore they couldn't possibly be allergic to it.

To begin with, very few of them succeeded in avoiding milk altogether since it occurs hidden in bread, biscuits, sausages and margarine, for example. The other point is that you have to *avoid enough foods to feel better* before you can infer that you were allergic to any. This will be explained to you in the course of this book and, indeed, is one of the many principles that you will need to learn to be fully *diet wise*!

Furthermore, if you do not allow yourself a sufficient amount of time away from the food before testing it you may get no obvious reaction, even from a bad allergy food when you return to it. This is probably the biggest single reason why so many people fail to detect their own allergies and why so many doctors are blind to the problem, especially in connection with food.

The reason is that you need to clear your bowel of the food before feeling any real benefits and definitely before testing it as a food challenge. That may take up to 5 days, or more if you are constipated. However there is a further complication, which is that if you wait *too long* before reintroducing a food, the reaction may settle down and not provoke any symptoms when you eat it as a test.

But allowing for these stumbling blocks, the definition holds good and is very workable: I have used it in my practice for many years now, often with spectacular results.

Non-immune allergens

To mainstream doctors, this concept would seem laughable or contradictory. But that doesn't mean they are correct in dismissing the idea. Many doctors said that anesthesia was impossible, heart transplants wouldn't work or that sunlight was not capable of curing rickets.

The fact is that we encounter the food allergy and intolerance problem often without any apparent immunological explanation. No antibodies show up. There has to be some other explanation than that the patient imagined it. For one thing, I have had countless reports over the years of patients reacting to a substance they were not even aware they were eating (hidden ingredients), so the phenomenon is real enough.

Note that von Pirquet's original definition did not require the antigen-antibody model. It had not even been discovered at the time.

In my era we still had not learned about the importance of genetic make up, though I was teaching the significance of individual biological variation. Nowadays this is coming to the fore and explains a great deal of the mechanism of food incompatibility.

US pioneers in allergy discoveries

After von Pirquet, a great deal of pioneer work in this field was begun right here in America. All those who practice it today have cause to be grateful to Dr. Albert Rowe Sr., who first experimented with elimination dieting in the 1920s. Following him came Dr. Herbert Rinkel, who verified the existence of the masked or hidden allergy, which I rate as one of the biggest medical discoveries since anesthetics and on a par with antibiotics; and who showed us how to rotate and diversify diets (see Chapter 15). Probably the greatest and most revered worker in the field, the doyen of environmental medicine, was the late Dr. Théron Randolph of Chicago (1906- 1995).

For years Randolph had to endure the scorn and reprobation of his colleagues: a story of courage and determination full of the very essence of human drama. Yet he persisted and saw his life's work vindicated. His book *Human Ecology and Susceptibility to the Chemical Environment* has become a classic text, and any doctor who has not read it should feel ashamed. Through his continued writings Randolph was probably our greatest voice; yet withal he continued to be an active clinician and researcher, well into his eighth decade. Other key names, all American, are Doris Rapp (already mentioned), William Rea, Michael Zeller, William Philpott, William Crook and Marshall Mandell.

Doctor Mac

In my old stomping ground in Britain, Dr. Richard Mackarness flew the flag for us and became a world-renowned name. He began as a consultant psychiatrist at the Park-Prewett Hospital in Basingstoke and, like many of his counterparts from across the Atlantic, took an interest in clinical ecology because he personally was a sufferer. Excluding certain foods helped him to a new life, and he realized it could do the same for others.

Of course he was scorned by his colleagues and probably had a tougher time than me, in the sense that I had little interest in what the die-hards at my local hospital believed, one way or the other. But Mackarness had to work in an intensely hostile environment of toxic psychiatry, supercilious arrogance and hospital food.

After a long and fruitful career and several international best-sellers, Mackarness retired to Australia, where he passed away. But his influence will continue for many years to come and his two main allergy books, *Not all in the Mind* and *Chemical Victims,* continue to command respect.

The Cambridge Group

There have now been stirrings in the scientific literature, it is true. Reports of two creditable studies have been published in *The Lancet,* the highly respected medical scientific journal. (Regrettably, most doctors are not in the habit of trying things for themselves and won't believe anything that hasn't been "proved" by a study that is published in a leading journal.) The first of these (November 20, 1982) has become known as "the Cambridge Study." Doctors Alan Jones, McLaughlin, Shorthouse, Workman and Hunter, working at Addenbrooks Hospital and the University of Cambridge showed that foods were able to provoke the symptoms of so-called irritable bowel syndrome in fourteen out of twenty-one patients. This was done double-blind, which means that extraneous factors, due perhaps to the patient knowing what he was being tested with, were ruled out. Irritable bowel syndrome is typical of many "mysterious" complaints which have kept conventional doctors puzzled for years. In actual fact, clinical ecologists have been saying it was food allergy for decades.

An even more historic step was the publication (October 1983) of the findings of a carefully staged study of migraine in children. Doctors Egger, Carter, Wilson and Turner and Professor Soothil of the Hospital for Sick Children and Institute of Child Care, Great Ormond Street, London, studied eighty-eight youngsters so afflicted. They were able to demonstrate a clear relationship with food and food additives in no fewer than eighty-two of those cases! Quite startling evidence, and very satisfying for alternative allergy physicians, who have had to bear their colleagues' scorn and indifference while trying to make it known that food and chemical allergies are by far the greatest factor in migraines.

Since then the trickle of studies has grown into a torrent. Yet still doctors are reluctant to accept that what we eat can have profound effects on our health. A seven-pound infant is entirely the result of nutrients supplied by the mother; a ten-stone (140 pound) adult is the product of whatever he or she has swallowed while growing up – yet still they don't seem to get it!

Arthur Coca's one-man allergy revolution

Before concluding this brief historical interlude, mention must be made of one key figure: Arthur F. Coca, MD (1875-1959). He was a very special physician, who managed to bridge alternative and mainstream medicine.

He gave us the important term *atopy*, meaning "strange disease." Coca also tried to introduce the word *'idioblapsis,'* which fortunately did not catch on.

Coca is best remembered for his pulse test technique. But in this context his most important contribution is in defining the issues. Although he was well-versed in immunology, indeed he was Professor of Immunology at Cornell University and founder of the Journal of Immunology, which he edited for thirty-two years, he clearly saw the standard immunological mechanisms were not the mechanisms by which most food allergy took place. Coca christened it "non-reaginic" food allergy (an antibody would be a reagin). He also noticed that troubles tended to run in families. So his full description for the phenomenon we shall be exploring in this book he called "familial non-reaginic food allergy."

We shall make some adaptation of his pulse method later in the book, when we come to food challenge tests.

6

Introducing the Basic Elimination Concept

Just how common are allergies and intolerance? Did our ancestors have them? These are questions I am often asked. The answer to the first can be simply put: there are many individuals who have a few allergies and a few individuals who have many allergies. It is the latter group who tend to become ill, and most of my patients belong to it. But if you cared to stop people in the street at random and questioned them closely enough, most of them would be able to report at least one food that disagreed with them in some way, whether so slightly as to cause no more than flatulence or badly enough to cause vomiting. If the problem is a very minor one and general health is good, few people give such reactions a second thought; they are considered almost 'normal.' The answer to the second question will take a little longer.

To understand this more fully it is necessary to inquire into what we should eat. Dr. Richard Mackarness, in his 1976 book *Not all in the Mind* , called our attention to the archaeological view of diet. Since then a number of authors have published on this theme, most notably S. Boyd Eaton MD, Marjorie Shostak and Melvin Konnor MD PhD, [*The Paleolithic Prescription*, Harper and Row, New York, 1988]. Konnor is an anthropologist MD and in a very strong position to comment regarding what our ancestors ate.

A little study in this direction suggests that primitive man's natural foods were fruit, vegetables and – when he could get them – meat or fish. This is called a "hunter-gatherer" subsistence. Incidentally, the joke is somewhat on the men: the big hunters, feeding the tribe – a testosterone-soaked archetype we are all familiar with. It turns out that over 60% of the calories consumed by Stone Age man were gathered by the women, just humble nuts, berries and seeds!

I myself did a little research while I lived in Sri Lanka. I was fascinated by the Balangodans, an Asian Cro-Magnon man. Archeological investigations, at several cave-dwelling sites, using accurate modern dating techniques, have shown continuous habitation there by the earliest modern Homo sapiens taking place for over 37,000 years. Cro-Magnon Man (*Homo sapiens sapientis*, the wisest of the wise) may have come out of Sri Lanka and not "out of Africa" at all! Known locally as the "Balangoda Man," after the district of the same name, these were very sophisticated people. Their fine microlithic tools pre-dated comparable artifacts of central Europe by almost 20,000 years. From skeletal evidence they were a very healthy lot, averaged almost 6 feet in height (174 cm.) and often lived to a great age. Balangodans ate a diet of plants, animals and seafood (oysters, molluscs and other gastropoda), typical of today's fashionable "detox" plans.

Farmer foods are unnatural

In Stone Age times there were no cereal products such as bread (from wheat); dairy produce was unknown beyond infancy; and stimulant drinks (such as tea and coffee), sugar and other modern foods of course did not form part of this very healthy diet. We are not programmed by genes to deal with these items.

Yet today we consume predominantly cereal foods (bread, cakes, cookies, pastry, and so on), dairy produce (milk, butter, cream, cheese and yoghurt), sugar, eggs and stimulant drinks, which do not belong in Man's diet and are therefore unnatural, whatever you may have heard to the contrary. I call these "farmer foods" and they have been in our diet only since the development of agriculture around 10,000 years ago; this is a blink of the eye in evolutionary terms. It would therefore not be surprising if eating as we do tended to cause ill health. Adverse reactions to foods would occur in direct proportion to the level of farmer foods in our diet, and that seems to be precisely what has happened: the less 'biological' food we eat, such as meat, fruit and vegetables, the more illness we are prone to.

The grass family

Grains are probably the worst offenders (biological classification *Graminacaea*): foods such as wheat, corn, rye, oats and barley (note buckwheat is not in this family of foods, see appendix A). Even the poet Chaucer referred to "blakke bread" as a cause of depression; that was probably made from rye in his day. Wheat is probably the number one allergy or intolerance food across the boards. Yet the propaganda runs high that wheat is a fine natural food. It isn't, as you can now understand.

Gluten enteropathy (celiac disease) is only a small part of this, despite the fact that around 1.5 million Americans now suffer from celiac disease (gluten allergy). The majority of patients I found, even those who felt well on a gluten-free regime, were not really gluten-sensitive but could eat one or more of the other gluten-containing foods (the four gluten foods are wheat, barley, rye and oats). In other words, for the vast majority, it is a wheat sensitivity, not a gluten sensitivity.

I have an even more contentious observation to point out to those steeped in false science: many patients report that they can eat white bread but cannot tolerate wholemeal. This is not quite as paradoxical as it first sounds: white bread is little more than powdered fluff, with the "wheatiness" refined out of it. Only eating the whole grain product brings on symptoms. While there are certain helpful nutrients in wheat germ, it can hardly be a safe food for those who are made ill by it.

Just another reverse-truth discovered by actual observation, not theories.

Milk is poison

Milk is another diet impostor. To listen to all the propaganda you would get the impression that anyone who didn't drink at least a pint of it a day was inevitably doomed to ill health. In fact, the opposite is probably true: millions of humans drink no milk at all and experience no deficiencies as a result, but a great many are made sick, without knowing it, by a milk allergy and intolerance. Children suffer particularly in this respect. Pumped full of milk to 'do them good', many are victims of severe milk allergy and so are constantly poorly with sore throats, runny noses, earache, 'teething troubles,' colic and a whole host of other childhood complaints which magically disappear when that substance is removed from their diet. The fact is that milk is not a natural food: no animal in nature drinks milk after its infancy, and it is completely illogical to suppose that Man must be different.

The idea that we need milk for calcium is no more than marketing propaganda. Consider this simple demographic: the USA, which has the highest consumption of dairy products in the world, has the highest incidence of osteoporosis. More women die of age-fracture of the femur than die of breast cancer. While the Chinese, traditionally entirely dairy-free, had no knowledge of osteoporosis. Once again, it is not genetic – Chinese women who switch to our Western diet begin to develop osteoporosis very rapidly. This is not hard to grasp if you understand that osteoporosis is a nutritional disease, not simply a lack of calcium. Magnesium and boron are actually far more valuable than calcium in promoting strong bones (400 mgm and 3 mgm daily, respectively).

If you pause to think for a moment you will realize that grains, dairy food and other farm produce such as eggs have only been in our diet since we settled the land and became civilized. Whereas there are many who would argue that civilization has not yet arrived, scholars would date this only from about ten thousand years ago – far more recently than you would think. In biology, where evolutionary changes take place slowly over millions of years, such a short time span is a drop in the ocean. In other words, we simply haven't had time to adapt to these new foodstuffs and as a result don't handle them well on ingestion. They are still alien foods so far as the cells of our body are concerned: our palate may be in the twentieth century, but our constitution is still that of a forest-dwelling higher ape. (This may be shocking to dedicated gourmets!)

The adulteration of food

But we have been eating cereals and milk for centuries, you say. True. And probably this has enabled most of us to tolerate such foods, all other things being equal. But additional factors have now been brought into the equation. Look at what has been happening to food in the last fifty years, especially the last twenty-five: now we have chemical food additives. Most of these have come into use only since the last World War, yet in just a few decades this adulteration of our basic foods has reached absurd proportions. Take a walk round any supermarket and look at the products on the shelves: it is almost impossible to buy simple, plain food. There are added colorants, emulsifiers, preservatives, flavor enhancers and scores of other alien ingredients that no one has had time to adapt to.

But before we consider those in a little more detail, do remember toxic substances, such as insecticides and fertilizers, that are sprayed onto crops before harvesting and eating and chemicals administered to livestock before slaughter for meat. There is a vast array of chemicals in the armament of the modern farmer or market gardener, almost all of which are as inimical to human life as they are to six-legged forms.

One of my patients was a farmer's wife, and she told me that she and her family wouldn't dream of eating the food they send to market for others to consume. "It's poisoned!" she declared, and she should know, since she and her husband were only too well aware of the abuses concerned. Instead, they grew their own food in a special plot without using chemicals. Like many farmers, they felt a keen economic pressure to use artificial methods to increase their yield. The irony of this is that 'organic' farming methods have been researched and advanced to the point where there is no long-term advantage in using chemicals.

Should I eat organic?

Unfortunately, organic eating remains expensive and ethical products are not always easy to obtain. The picture is now complicated by persistent lobbying by unethical food producers, who have succeeded in getting the laws changed to redefine "organic" as something fake, which suits their wily purposes. Fortunately, I have got the majority of my patients well eating normal commercial supplies of foodstuffs. It is unquestionably more convenient.

To be really safe is a very complex issue and I find that it becomes somewhat overwhelming for the average individual. Did you know for example, that ethylene (a toxic chemical gas used in blowtorches) is used to force the ripening of apples, bananas and tomatoes? The gas of course contaminates the crop, but would never be listed as an ingredient or a contaminant. The rules simple don't require it. Most people know that wax is sprayed onto the skin of apples and other fruit to make them more attractive. But did you know many foods are treated with sulfites before being cooked? Again this is not an "ingredient" as such and so you, the consumer, are not going to be warned.

Then there is the whole problem surrounding the safety of genetically-modified foods. Unfortunately, that is beyond the scope of this book.

But there are other concerns too, like mercury contamination of fish stocks, which is now, frankly, quite worrying.

These issues spill over into politics and go beyond personal health imperatives. Be alert to the spin and lies from fake watchdogs like Consumer Alert, which claims to be a consumer advocacy group but is really an industry lobby group that campaigns against consumer rights – such as the right to have GM food labeled. It opposes organic farming, DDT regulation and the Kyoto treaty. (It is funded by the tobacco industry and other socially-irresponsible corporations.)

Food additives

The real long-term health concern is deliberate additives to processed and manufactured foods. When I first started writing about diet issues in the early 80s, I frequently had to point out that food allergy and intolerance was not simply a matter of "junk food" or, as people usually supposed, food additives and flavorings to alter the taste of food. These include MSG and what is laughably called natural flavoring are used to artificially enhance the taste of food so that it tastes better. In other words their sole purpose is to sell you stuff you wouldn't otherwise eat it. Trust me.

Be especially aware of hydrolyzed vegetable protein, which is sometimes passed off as "natural flavorings," since it comes from vegetables. You should know that the vegetables are treated with an acid soak, followed by caustic soda to neutralize the acid. The end result is a brown sludge that you are expected to believe is "natural." Other ingredients to look out for are vegetable protein, textured protein, hydrolyzed plant protein, soy protein extract, caseinate and yeast extract.

These disgusting products are added to a huge variety of foods, from canned tuna to baby food. Yes, baby food! This is despite the fact that it is known that the immature nervous system is especially vulnerable to these bandit food ingredients. Don't get fooled by the quantities either, or believe they are safe. There is enough monosodium glutamate in a single bowl of commercially available soup to raise a child's blood glutamate beyond that required to cause nerve damage in immature animals.

One of the MSG industry's chief arguments for the safety of their product is that glutamate in the blood cannot cross the so-called blood-brain barrier. This is incorrect. Parts of the brain are not protected by the blood-brain barrier and one of the most important, the hypothalamus, is especially susceptible to damage by glutamate in MSG.

One of the earliest and most consistent findings with exposure to MSG is damage to an area of the hypothalamus known as the arcuate nucleus. This small group of special cells controls a multitude of neuroendocrine functions, as well as being intimately connected to several other hypothalamic nuclei, to which the malfunction will spread.

In any case there are many disorders known to alter the permeability of the blood-brain barrier and cause it to "leak." These conditions include hypertension, diabetes, ministrokes, major strokes, head trauma, multiple sclerosis, brain tumors, chemotherapy, radiation treatments to the nervous system, collagen-vascular diseases (lupus), AIDS, brain infections, a number of drugs and Alzheimer's disease. Moreover the blood-brain barrier protects less and less as a consequence of natural aging. There may be many other conditions also associated with barrier disruption that are as yet not known.

Fore more information, I refer you to Russell Blaylock's excellent book *EXCITOTOXINS: The Taste That Kills*, Health Press, Santa Fe, 1997.

Vitiation of foods

Vitiation means weakening or reducing the worth of. Food which has undergone this process of degradation we call junk food. Ironically, some people with pronounced allergies or intolerance can get away with eating junk foods. That's a sign of just how little real food there is present.

But such foods do nothing to build real health and combat disease. Today we are seeing a new kind of malnutrition in the West. It isn't caused by low calorie intake, as in the old days, but by lack of nutritious ingredients. People are eating bulk and not quality. The present epidemic of obesity seen in the USA is as much about eating the wrong food as eating too much food. Those of you who have trouble relating to what you read in a book should rent a copy of Milton Spurlock's movie *Super Size Me* and watch it.

Spurlock conducted an experiment on himself, which he documented with film footage, to measure the health impact of eating three meals a day for thirty days at McDonald's. He gained twenty-five pounds. Worse than that: within a few days of beginning his diet of cheeseburgers, fried and chocolate shakes, Spurlock, a healthy thirty-three-year old, was vomiting out the window of his car, and doctors who examined him were shocked at how rapidly Spurlock's entire body deteriorated. His liver became toxic, his cholesterol shot up from a low 165 to 230, his libido flagged and he suffered headaches and depression.

"It was really crazy – my body basically fell apart over the course of thirty days," Spurlock reported to the press.

Predictably, no one from Macdonald's would comment.

A frightening experiment on the effects of vitiated food

In the first edition of this book I reported on a far earlier study of the effects of vitiated foodstuffs. This time it was on animals, cats actually; so there was no possibility of human reactions and emotions clouding the picture.

Between 1932 and 1942 Dr. Francis M. Pottenger conducted a number of nutritional experiments on domestic cats. Certain animals were put on diets consisting only of pasteurized milk and cooked meats, equivalent to our processed or junk foods and quite unlike the normal, healthy cat diet of raw meat. Predictably, the animals became ill, antisocial, aggressive and exhibited deviant sexual behavior. By the third generation these cats were so effete as to be sterile, so that those particular strains died out. Even soy beans planted in the floor of the cages housing the affected animals failed to sprout, whereas the same plants grew happily and flourished in the cages with the controls fed on raw foods.

But what was really disturbing was the fact that cats taken off the deficient diet took three generations to return to normal health parameters. The cats were eating foods in total violation of their nutritional genomics and the results of that were disastrous in the long term.

Parallels with our modern human diets are inevitable, and if the findings hold true for us as well as for cats, the implications are very serious indeed: namely that through bad eating we are ruining not only our own health but also that of our children and grandchildren. What cannot be argued is that antisocial behavior (measured as crime) has gotten worse, educational standards have fallen and sperm counts have dropped. Could all this be linked to bad diet?

I say yes.

Unfortunately, this very important study has gone largely ignored by the medical establishment. There are several reasons for this: to begin with, the medical profession as a whole tends to ignore nutrition as being relevant to health; secondly, although this experiment was a milestone and undoubtedly years ahead of its time, it failed to conform to current criteria in medical scientific rhetoric.

What cooking does to food

There is one last issue I want to address on the topic of altered foodstuffs and that is the question of cooking. Heat changes food chemically, often for the worse. But sometimes for better too.

Let me explain this apparently strange remark.

We know that heat changes chemicals and denatures protein, one of the chief food classes we eat. For example, the reason that egg "white" turns from clear into opaque white is that its albumin, a kind of protein, has been denatured. This renders it worthless nutritionally; but we don't care much because most of the nutrients of use to chicks and humans is in the yolk, which is thus best left runny.

Heat also inactivates enzymes and gets rid of most vitamin content. This is not good for nutrition and, quite rightly, there is an interest in eating raw food. We should consume plenty.

However, a surprising number of foods are toxic in their natural state, as I detailed in chapter 2. Heating may render them edible. For instance, red kidney beans need to be cooked really well, otherwise they tend to cause bellyache. Many other pulses (peas and beans) are also toxic for humans;

the lathyrus bean (Lathyrus sativus) causes lathyrism, a permanent nerve paralysis. When crops fail in Asia, starving people sow the bean and use it to feed themselves but the result is a tragic outbreak of paraplegia. Naturally occurring poisons that mimic organophosphates (developed as nerve gas by the Nazis in World War II) are known to occur in plants of the genus Solanum, which includes potatoes, tomatoes, and eggplants. Poisoning has resulted from ingestion of potato sprouts, sprouted potatoes, and greened potatoes. Symptoms of green potato poisoning include stomach pain, nausea and vomiting, rapid and difficult respiration, and death. The humble carrot also contains a nerve toxin. As someone joked, even the cabbage, if it was subjected to safety tests such as drugs are subjected to, it would not pass!

The fact is that many foods are toxic and we humans could not normally eat them. Thorough cooking destroys most of the toxin (but not all allergenicity), and A. C. Leopold and R. Arthrey have pointed out that it is probably only since the advent of fire that man has been able to eat a number of foods which are inherently toxic (Leopold, A. C. & Ardrey, R. "Toxic substances in plants and food habits in Early Man, " *Science*, 176, 512, 1972).

Historically, primitive Man's conquest of his environment began as a result of his being able to eat a much wider diet and so being able to increase in terms of numbers which could be supported by a given acreage. Fire (and cooking) may be the real reason for our mastery of the Earth and not just tools, as is commonly supposed. These are interesting anthropological speculations, and they put the enormous value of the discovery of fire into perspective for us. If the theory is correct, it would mean that pulses, like cereals and dairy produce, are relatively new food substances for us and that we have not had long in which to adapt to them.

Remember this section when you encounter the persuasions of total raw food enthusiasts.

Meantime, this is an allergy doctor telling you cook most food reasonably. Do not overcook, because the browning effect which is produced contains acrylamides. These substances are also nerve toxins and, by the way, thought to be carcinogenic. Eat plenty of raw foods, especially greens and fruit; you need the antioxidants and enzymes.

But remember, this book is different: nothing in general overrides the fact that your own tolerances are unique. Whatever we establish, later in the book, is bad for you, you must not eat.

Back to the caveman diet

By now you may be wondering if you are someone who could benefit from the diet plan in this book. If you feel less than vibrant and anticipate each new day with less than enthusiasm, not to mention if you have symptoms that no doctor has been, to date, able to cure, then I urge you to keep reading.

Of course, you won't know for sure if this diet plan is for you until and unless you try it. However, in my quarter of a century of clinical experience, I learned that these diet principles work for everybody.

Later we'll be using a trial diet – a diet much like what cavemen and women would have eaten, to test for the possibilities of food allergy and intolerance. The so-called Stone Age diet consists of meat, fish, fruit and vegetables, with water to drink (herb teas are allowed). It's quite enjoyable, since you are allowed fries, fish, steak, smoothies and other familiar foods. It's not a slimming diet and you are free to eat as much as you like; there is no reason to be hungry on this plan.

It is important to understand this is a trial diet – a test. You do not need to stay on such a strict diet. As soon as symptoms clear, we then begin challenge testing, to find out the real culprits. These few foods will be the only ones that you need to avoid long-term. In other words your maintenance diet is different from the trial diet. I do not encourage anyone to try to remain on the strict Stone Age diet. Moreover, it isn't logical. If you give up a score of foods and feel better, that doesn't mean that all were to blame. It may be just one or two foods that are the real culprits.

What happens if I'm allergic to the allowed foods?

I'm sure you will be aware that some people are allergic to meat, some to fruit and so on. This is not a zero-allergy diet. It's simply playing the odds. Because these are our natural foods, the ones we should be eating, they are better tolerated and therefore less likely to provoke symptoms, as I have explained. I'm asking you to give up the most likely foods for a few days.

If it emerges that you are allergic to meat or other allowed foods, we will still get a result and you will be shown how to test for this. Chapter 12 has all the details.

But before we get to the *how*-to, let's look at a little more *why*.

7

The Hidden, or "Masking" Effect Explained

L et me say a little more about the mechanism of disguised allergy, as it applies to food as well as to other allergies.

A significant light was shed by Herbert Rinkel MD, an American doctor who has made a great contribution to medical science in the 1930s and 40s. Rinkel discovered himself to be allergic to eggs despite eating large quantities of them on a virtually daily basis. (When Rinkel was an indigent student, his father, who was a farmer, kept him well supplied with eggs for years.) Rinkel suffered from severe catarrh, but when the supply of eggs was temporarily interrupted for a few days, the catarrh cleared up dramatically! Rinkel immediately suspected an egg reaction; but the clinch came when he next ate an egg as a test. He passed out!

From these clues, Rinkel was able to reason out the mechanism involved: *repeated ingestion of the food was somehow damping down the reaction, so that there was no obvious connection between the symptoms and the intake of a particular food.* Here was yet another case of a chance observation grasped upon by a brilliant mind which comprehends significances that most ordinary people would pass by. An understanding of exactly how a hidden allergy or intolerance works is of vital importance to you in solving your own case. The explanation that follows is given in terms of food allergy and genetic food intolerance, but it is important to remember that the same principles apply to chemicals, dust, molds and other sensitivities as well.

Suppose you are allergic to milk and dairy produce (it happens to be a very common allergy) and ate it almost every day: cereals with milk for breakfast each morning; milk with coffee or tea, perhaps. Your body would adapt in an unhappy fashion to this daily onslaught of toxin.

For long periods you might feel quite well; then you have a sudden attack of your complaint. You would say to yourself, not unreasonably: 'It can't be milk. I ate it last week *and* the week before and I didn't have any symptoms!' But if this was a *hidden* allergy you would be quite wrong: that's exactly how it could behave. Perhaps you might become suspicious of milk and decide to have a glass of milk, just to see if you can prove you are sensitive to it. Nothing happens. You might even have your best day for weeks. It's all very baffling, and not surprisingly it was a long while before this mechanism was fully understood; even now it defeats the careless or casual observer. It simply doesn't work to 'eat something and see.'

Unless you have the knowledge I am going to share with you in this book, you might never uncover this mechanism.

Frequency is the pointer

To start with, there are two very useful clues which point the way to what we are looking for. In order for an allergy or genetic incompatibility to hide or mask, the victim must eat the food with a certain minimum frequency. By experience I find this to be about twice a week, though the exact interval varies from person to person.

If you ate the culprit food only occasionally, you would have your attack only once in a while and the chances are it wouldn't take you long to work out what was happening. This is precisely the reason allergies to strawberries or shellfish are so notorious: most of us eat these foods only a few times a year. The body doesn't get the chance to develop a hidden allergy, so there is never any doubt about the severity of the reaction. The real troublemakers are foods eaten frequently, often daily. It is as if the body learns to cope with the problem, and we sometimes speak of becoming 'adapted' to an allergen. 'Maladapted' is the opposite and denotes the periods when it makes you unavoidably ill.

The reason twice a week is an important interval in masking an allergy from view has to do with bowel habit. It takes about four days, on average, to empty the bowel, and if a food is eaten more frequently this means it is *permanently within the body*. People vary, of course. For someone with chronic diarrhea, the interval may be shorter; constipation, on the other hand, increases it. In other words, there is always some of the food present in the bowel, so a further intake may not provoke any overt symptoms.

Addiction

The second *big* clue I have already mentioned is that patients tend to get hooked on their allergens (allergen: a substance which causes an allergy reaction). This is an aspect of the problem that intrigues patients and public alike. I'm talking now about real addiction: if the patient goes too long without that food or substance, symptoms begin which induce a craving. More of the food puts an end to the symptoms temporarily, and the craving ceases for a time.

Thus the food or drink appears to give a 'lift,' but you must understand that this is only because it is causing a 'down' in the first place. You may know someone who always feels better for a cup of tea or a cookie; it is possible to see such people visibly perk up. That's addiction at work, and, I need hardly point out, it is very common! The mechanism is in no way different from the addiction of a junkie to heroin, or of an alcoholic to liquor. Neither, in certain cases, are the consequences any less drastic – it's just a socially more acceptable addiction, that's all.

Patients would say to me at the office, 'Doctor, I'll give up anything you say – as long as it isn't bread!' (for bread, read tea, sugar, milk, coffee, potatoes, and so on). Immediately, of course, I suspected that this was something they were going to *have* to give up in order to get well. Sometimes I was accused by my patients of being puritanical: to them it seems I was bent on stopping the things they enjoy and crave the most, and often they are right. Usually this was no more than a jocular criticism, but there were occasions when I was faced with raw, steamy emotion. I had to explain that it was not my fault the situation had come about; I merely had to treat the after-effect of years, even a lifetime, of wrong eating habits.

It is interesting to note in passing that migraine patients are told not to go more than a few hours without food. To do so often provokes an attack of migraine on you, dear reader, now you know why! But I find it baffling and frustrating that the doctors concerned, who are aware of its withdrawal effect, never make the mental leap to recognizing they are dealing with an *addiction*.

So what is a masked allergy or intolerance?

This addiction mechanism gives rise to another important new term, the *masked allergy*. Essentially, this is the same as a hidden allergy, but it reminds us that in this instance ingesting the allergen is what keeps the symptom at bay: in other words, it masks the withdrawal effect, provided it is eaten often enough. How often is enough? The interval can vary from as little as one or two hours to forty-eight hours or more; on rare occasions it can exceed seventy-two hours. Remember that if you suffer from constipation or diarrhea these intervals can vary up or down. I have seen patients who start getting a headache and feeling depressed if they don't get a cup of coffee every couple of hours or so – just look at some of the people in the queue at Starbuck's! You'll see plenty of tense faces and irritable body language!

Now you may understand the very common experience: that of feeling pretty rough first thing in the morning. Many people wake tired and irritable and are slow to start their day. It seems that until they have eaten breakfast, they behave like a bear with a sore head. Well, by the time we awake, many of us have been off food some 10 – 14 hours. That's easily enough to set up withdrawal symptoms. *That oh-so common feeling is a classic diagnostic sign of one or more hidden allergies.*

The victim eats some wheat (toast), corn (cereal), soaked with milk and sugar (two of the commonest culprits), and drinks a coffee or tea (caffeine); one or more of these fixes the withdrawal symptoms, winds up the individual to full capacity and off they go, fully restored for a working day. Or at least for a few hours, until they need some more coffee, a cookie, or whatever!

The proof of what I am sharing with you here is so easy to establish. You'll do it for yourself, following the plan in the book. When you give up the offending food or foods, you'll probably have some terrible withdrawals at first. But then, after about five days, you will end up bouncing out of bed with zest and hit the ground running each morning. Then you will know *for sure*, I'm right.

Selye's General Theory of Adaptation

These observed food masking effects are easy to explain, using Hans Selye's General Adaptation Syndrome (GAS for short). If you haven't read Selye's very capable book, *The Stress of Life*, you should. He postulates three stages in coping with stress. This progression would be exhibited by any organism in response to any form of stress, from an amoeba living in slightly tainted water all the way to a pressurized executive in a demanding, harassing job that is giving him ulcers.

At first the organism reacts strongly to the new unpleasant stimulus: it fights it, and it is this struggle that we recognize in terms of "symptoms."

In human terms, the organism would feel ill. Hippocrates called it the *ponos,* or strife, of disease, and without it no disease exists. Selye called it Stage 1.

Then, gradually, adaptation occurs. The organism learns to cope with the problem. The symptoms reduce or disappear, and the disease submerges; the human subject feels well again. Selye recognizes this as a separate development, or Stage 2. It *appears* that there are no further problems. Yet all the while an insidious attack is taking place. This steadily erodes the body's defenses until eventually they are exhausted. The process may take months or decades, but it advances inexorably as long as the stress is present. Finally, when the body can simply cope no more, symptoms reemerge, and this is Stage 3. The organism is sick, as before, but now in difficulties because there are no defenses left. This is the stage of chronic illness.

Following from the concept of adaptation, we can consider this new development to be *maladaptation,* which in my view would be a far better term than either allergy or intolerance. Maladaptation to foods is so common I consider it to be almost universal. Answer the questions honestly in the next chapter and you will begin to see what I mean!

Selye's General Adaptation Syndome is an attractive theory and fits many observations I have made among sick people. It also parallels very closely the histories of allergy or intolerance sufferers, which is why it is of special interest to us. Many people I question can remember being made ill by certain foods as children: their parents insisted they eat the foods because 'They are good for you.' In time the foods were tolerated (the person became adapted to them: Stage 2); but now, years later, the unlucky individual is sick with asthma, arthritis, migraine or any one of a host of diseases, and often we track down these very foods as being the cause of the problem. This is Stage 3, and the body has no resistance left so the condition is chronic. Incidentally, the mechanism of addiction to a food coincides with Stage 3: not only is the patient unable to oppose the food physically, but it is as if he or she is unable to oppose it mentally either and has to have it.

Stage 4 overload

Selye did not postulate a Stage 4 but I am adding to his theory here by suggesting that the masking step goes beyond Stage 3. In this additional aspect, which we can consider as a fourth stage, the food relieves the symptoms temporarily. But the patient is now on dangerous ground and the destructive results of the continued daily or hourly stress can cause a breakdown of almost any organ in the body.

Many of the symptoms, as we shall see, relate to mind and brain function and chronic fatigue, fuzzy thinking (which we call "woolly brain syndrome") and unpleasant moods are the norm for this final stage.

Stress overload

In support of the connection with Selye's GAS model, I can state that many allergy-based illnesses come on or get worse after periods of acute stress such as an episode of a severe infective disease, bereavement, divorce or redundancy. It is as if the extra burden becomes too great for the body, already under siege, which then moves rapidly from Stage 2 into Stage 3. While adapted, the body could cope – barely – but not in the face of extra stress.

Unfortunately, patients often do not recover once the stress is removed again; after the allergies or maladaptation have been triggered, so to speak, they cause illness in their own right. This disease is further stress, which causes further illness, and a vicious circle seems to come about with the result that the patient may still be ill *years* after, say, his or her father died, even though that was what seemed to have brought on the illness in the first place. This is important because it is a situation from which the only escape seems to be solving the allergies.

The final supportive evidence for Selye's theory working in this context is the following observation: *the more you eat of a food the more likely you are to develop a maladaptation to it.* Overeating a substance will cause it to disagree with you. The food itself becomes a stress and will accelerate Stage 3.

This is almost certainly the reason why wheat, milk, sugar and so on are such common food allergies. Not only are they not really 'natural' foods, which makes them stressful, but they are considerably over-consumed by the population as a whole. Most diets are heavily loaded with bread, milk, sweeteners and cereal products. This may suit the fast-food chains, but I doubt if Mother Nature is amused.

You will hear me say over and over in this book that repetitive eating causes food reactions.

Now the new genetic incompatibility theory

None of these empirical observations on stress and overload contradict the emergent science of nutritional genomics. In this model we know that certain foods are not tolerated because the individual lacks genes which provide metabolic pathways for disposing of chemical substances making up the food (remember the outline of the many toxins that are to be found in food, pages 18-22). There is also the backlash effect I mentioned early on in Chapter 1, where eating certain foods can bring on a gene reaction, whether good or bad.

We are all different. You take after your parents somewhat, but you are unique because some of your genes will manifest and others will not (we call this gene "expression").

That explains why some people feel good on a particular diet and others feel bad. The authors of these fad diets will not come clean and tell you this happens – patients who report problems are just looked on as freaks (or troublemakers). But now you know this is bound to happen. Cutting edge science says it must.

Ironically, this new specialty of nutritional genomics came about through studying idiosyncratic drug reactions. Some patients were being hurt and even killed by drugs which didn't seem to be threatening to the majority of us. Over 100,000 people are year are killed by adverse drug reactions in the US alone. Despite being diametrically opposed to the unscrupulous drug industry I am prepared to concede they don't *like* killing their customers, if only because it costs big money and creates insurance problems. But in fact the investigation of why some individuals respond in a dramatically different way to the same substance led to the discovery of the important of gene-mediated metabolic pathways.

Personalized medicine

We will soon all be speaking of what may be termed "personalized medicine."

The time will come when we will all be routinely tested for our genomic profile and advised accordingly what substances (foods and chemicals) are safe for us and what we should avoid. HRT may be great for some women but drive others inexorably towards cancer and heart disease; beta carotene may protect some people against cancer but can cause it in others; vitamin A, taken as an immune booster can increase the chance of susceptible women getting a hip fracture; decreasing blood homocysteine levels with B vitamins actually causes more fatal heart conditions, despite lowering the homocysteine levels; and so it goes on... Without the correct gene profile in hand, doctors are, in effect, merely guessing which drugs to administer and running a lottery on which patients will die and which will live.

It's going to change! In fact I can tell you the FDA is taking a direct interest in enforcing the practice of personalized medicine. You might be a little cynical about the FDA's record in protecting people from the drug industry. But this move is bound to be a big step forward in curbing reckless and dangerous prescribing. The time will come when conventional doctors will be investigating what is different about you instead of insisting that you are merely average and like everyone else on Earth. The FDA is calling these tests multivariate index assays; guidelines were issued March 22, 2005.

8

Overload and Target Organs

Y ou sneezed, you feel achy. There, another sneeze. You've got 'flu, right?

Most likely wrong. One of the commonest symptoms I encountered in my clinical working years was a bunch of symptoms which suggested 'flu but which wasn't. In fact the patient was sometimes well again next day. A viral infection doesn't clear like that; ten days to mount a full immune response, more likely.

Think about what you already know. What is the commonest cliché for an allergy? A sneeze! So a bout of sneezing could be an allergy, just as surely as it might mean an upper respiratory infection. If you add aches and pains that still doesn't mean 'flu. Only if there is a fever should 'flu be your first suspicion and that is, frankly, quite rare.

Many people suffer bouts of colds or 'flu but which clear up in 24 - 72 hours. These are not infections but allergic reactions and are very common, once you know what to look for. Do not be fooled into thinking that only inhaled allergens affect the airways; *you do not have to breathe the allergen to get respiratory symptoms*. In fact one of the most important things I discovered in all those years I practiced was that 85% or more of respiratory allergy, asthma included, was because of food reactions.

Even if the patient is allergic to dust and house mites, this is often secondary. Because a person reacts strongly to dust and dust mites does not mean that these are the causative agents of asthma or rhinitis.

The real culprit I found, time and time again, was one or more foods. I found this because I did not quit at the first diagnostic clue but went all the way. I have seen many hundreds of cases where a person was allergic to dust yet when they changed their diet, they made a substantial recovery.

This accords very well with Selye's GAS theory. Reducing the overall load helps the person recover and he or she will move back from

Stage 3 to Stage 2; that is, from maladaptation to once again adapted. Hey presto, the symptoms disappear!

No more hay fever!

I took this one simple technique and used it successfully over and over, in situations where it was not easy to avoid a key allergen but dietary change is always possible. Consider the annual bugaboo of hay fever. We all know this is caused by reactions to pollen, tiny plant grains floating in the air. Many patients lead miserable restricted lives throughout the best months of the year because they cannot go outdoors without suffering severely from runny nose and reddened, itchy eyes.

I used my ingenuity and knowledge of the GAS theory to engineer a solution which worked for most sufferers, which was to implement a change of diet during the peak summer months. Hay fever (from grass) is caused by allergy to grass pollen; so I had patients stop eating grass! Most people looked startled at the idea and protested they don't eat grass. Women particularly, sometimes glared at me as if I were calling them a cow. But the truth is we all eat grasses or grains: wheat (bread, cakes, cookies, muffins, pastry, pasta etc), corn (polenta, hominy, grits, etc.), oatmeal, rice and rye are all foods from the grass family.

It is logical that stopping eating large quantities of grass will allow a greater tolerance of the inhaled grass pollen grains and, sure enough, it worked. Pretty soon my story was leaked to the media and every spring and summer for the next decade I was called up by press and radio from all over the world to repeat this wonderful healing trick for the benefit of their readers and listeners. Giving up bread, pasta and such foods was a lot less stressful than being miserable and unable to go outdoors for weeks at a time. Many patients, even taking antihistamines, were not able to lead a normal life, until they tried the Scott-Mumby diet solution!

Of course not all hay fever is caused by grass pollens. Tree pollen, flowers, shrubs and even circulating mold spores can have the same effect. But the diet trick still worked just the same. Some individuals who are sensitive to ragweed may also react to melon and cantaloupe and would be better to give it up for the "season." That's because it all comes down to body load, and any legitimate means of reducing the body's burden will reduce the pressure on its defenses.

Pretty soon I came to realize that any kind of unburdening helped and a good general low-allergy diet, such as the one described in these pages, would bring relief for those few critical weeks. Try it yourself next season, if you suffer from hay fever.

Any food, any symptom

I'm saying all that to make a very important point which is that any food (or indeed any stressor) can impact any part of the body or any organ. The symptoms which result have little or no relevance, contrary to the way most doctors look at this. All through med school, trainee doctors are taught to look for combinations of symptoms, called a syndrome or "disease," which is a fixed pattern of ailments that recurs each time. This helps to identify the supposed cause. Thus a certain kind of respiratory distress in which exhalation of breath is difficult and accompanied by wheezing sounds, often provoked by dust and sometimes by emotions, is called *asthma*. For a doctor that fixes it and the correct drugs are prescribed.

But it says nothing about the real cause of this problem. Often it is known that inhalant allergies cause provocation. But sometimes this is not the case and doctors are then baffled. They have never done the years of trial and error that I did and proven to themselves, as I have, that over 85% or asthma is food allergy or genetic food intolerance and on a correctly maintained diet, excluding the patients' allergens, most will recover completely.

Casebook 3.

One of my early cases was Mark, a young boy of fourteen. He was what we call a "respiratory cripple": his lungs were so bad at oxygenating the blood that he could hardly walk. Mark was just as much a cripple as if he'd had a withered leg. Just to get by he needed oxygen several times a day; that meant he could not go to school and had to study at home, with his oxygen tank on hand. Mark was also taking, as I remember, around seven or eight different medications.

The fact that the meds were clearly of no value did not stop his regular physician from prescribing these toxins. In fact when the boy relapsed and symptoms got worse, that was taken as a sign to increase the doses he was taking. Not very logical in my view. People in this precarious mode of existence often die due to one final severe asthma attack. The drugs are already pushed to the limit and therefore there is nothing left with which to bring the patient out of the crisis. It is so needless: the patient is not suffering a drug deficiency, therefore drugs did not and could not solve the problem – only stall the symptoms somewhat.

Asthma, of course, is an inflammatory process (often made worse by stress and other factors). The most likely inflammation is an allergy. Most doctors think of dust and mold, arrange skin tests and then, when these prove negative, think no further of the allergy problem. Again, very defective logic. Even when dust or mite allergy show up, that may be misleading. The physician assumes this is the cause of the allergic inflammation and never looks any further. If the real culprit is a food and the patient is given the false and deadly belief that the cause of the problem is dust, he or she is left with a double whammy. Nothing is going to resolve the problem. A lifetime of medications – a short one at that – is on the cards for sure.

In Mark's case, he was lucky. I quickly found that dairy products and eggs were killer pathogens, I took him off the foods and he recovered quickly and completely. The last I heard of him was a nice letter from his Mum: Mark was attending college doing fine, enjoyed athletics and was in the rugby football team, playing forward (a fast runner position).

Think the allergens I keep listing are pretty much the same?

Luke was a 58-year-old man with severe asthma. He was so allergic to tomatoes he could not even tolerate their presence. Avoiding tomatoes, he was symptom-free. Then one day he was carrying home the groceries from the corner store and developed a severe wheezing attack. Luke was puzzled until he found that one of the bags he had been hugging to his chest contained tomatoes (his wife had arranged the grocery pick-up and forgot to warn him).

Overload

One of the most important of all healing principles, if not *the* most important, is that of *total body load*. It is the key to all recoveries and overcoming all disease processes. No doctor really cures anything; Nature does that. All the successful physician can do is to reduce body load to allow this process to take place. Unfortunately, modern medicine and its drugs often *adds* to the biological burden instead of relieving it.

Along with all living creatures we are endowed with a number of key regulatory mechanisms. One can only be amazed that they rarely seem to break down, rather than being surprised and disconcerted when they do. The skin protects us from temperature variation and dehydration, the immune system wards off micro-organisms, the kidneys eliminate poison waste, the liver detoxifies an ever-increasing amount of xenobiotic (alien) chemicals and other factors regulate the acid-base balance within the body. Every day, every minute, trouble is nipped in the bud before it gets started and we remain unaware of what is taking place: we feel OK. It is only when the defenses are overworked that we actually experience any health problems at all. By the time we are aware of a symptom, any symptom, the defenses have already broken down and matters are really quite serious.

Types of overload

Overloading the system is thus asking for trouble. This is true for all of us, not just allergy patients. There are many ways to overload. Table 11.1 summarizes most of these. A mere glance will tell you that this list is also a summary of clinical ecology to date.

Conditions Contributing to Overload:

Stress	Endocrine disorders
Allergies	Electromagnetic fields
Chemical pollution	Fatigue
Drugs	Nutritional deficiencies
Geopathic stress	Radioactivity
Mercury toxicity	Alcohol
Hidden infections	Oxidative stress

Overload can lead to an almost infinite variety of disease symptoms. Mental breakdown, heart disease, ulcers and cancer are just some of the possibilities. Which symptoms arise from which stressor comes under the consideration of so-called target (or 'shock') organs. Something will break down and usually it is the inherent weak link that snaps first. If the overload is prolonged or severe, more and more end-organs will fail and symptoms and complications will multiply.

Reducing the load

The opposite side of the equation works just as effectively and can be turned to good use by a skilled physician. Any legitimate means of reducing body load helps, directly or indirectly, with any illness: better nutrition will aid the fight against cancer; eating fewer stress foods can help hay fever (stress foods include those you are allergic to, refined carbohydrates – which can cause adrenal stress – or food additives [chemical toxins], etc.); clearing up hidden infections such as Candida will reduce PMT; eliminating hairsprays and perfumes may improve catarrh (even though dust is the main cause); stopping smoking aids fertility and moving away from geopathic stress will help alleviate almost any disease process. I'm on record with the BBC saying even a divorce might lead to a recovery!

Now you may understand why you can eat a food you are normally allergic to while on holiday (where your mental stress and, probably, the amount of chemical pollutions are far less) with no ill effects.

If you understand overload and work to avoid it this very important principle will serve you well.

Threshold values

Implicit in the overload theory is that the body has certain thresholds of tolerance. Only when these limits are exceeded will symptoms occur.

Bad allergens, then, are the ones of which even a tiny quantity puts you over the limit. Mild allergies are those which need a big dose of an allergen to come into effect. Probably mild allergies would not arise at all if the allergens were encountered in normal quantities, but several together can add up to trouble. It is even possible to imagine a scale and assign arbitrary numerical values. If your threshold limit is, say 10 points, a 12 allergy would put you straight into symptoms. But one or two 3s taken together would still have no effect; two 4s and a 3 might, and so on. This can be represented diagrammatically. (See figure below.)

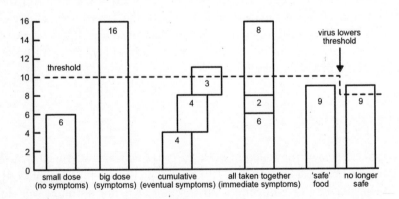

The 'values' scale may be a bit artificial but if you get the idea of allergies being cumulative, you will avoid unpleasant consequences more often. You will also begin to understand why sometimes you can eat a food without any effect and at other times be ill.

Why most people feel better on vacation

Incidental life events can play havoc with these threshold levels. Virus infections often shift the values markedly, usually to the patient's disadvantage; so does emotional stress. If bad things are happening in a person's life, I always counsel them to be much more careful than usual about what they eat. Of course the tendency, when under duress, is to do exactly the opposite and let standards fall. That's one reason why people become ill when under stress.

You will probably understand that this also applies in reverse. When you are relaxed and happy you can get away with eating indiscretions, whereas normally you would expect symptoms. That's one of the main reasons people feel better on holiday: their overload and intolerances recede and symptoms may disappear altogether.

Now you understand the mechanism! You see, when you learn the *real* reason for things, it all starts to make sense. You are truly becoming *diet wise*...

Just don't expect to get away with the same dietary excesses when you are back home!

Individual food overload

Time and again I will be advising you not to eat one food repetitively but to vary your intake. It is possible to think in terms of *individual food overload*. To eat one food in excess is really just another aspect of Selye's GAS hypothesis and will cause system stress. In its fullest format a rotation diet prevents the repetitive eating of any particular food but also guards against eating closely related foods too frequently. Not everyone, fortunately, needs to follow a strict rotation plan but variety in eating is a key health principle. This will be explained in Chapter 15.

Target organs

The final and most interesting aspect of the overload model is that of "target" or "shock" organs. I have referred to this several times already. When the body is stressed, as with bandit foods that cause trouble, the overload phenomenon comes into play. But the exact symptoms that manifest depend on what part of the body or what organ system gets hit most.

We doctors also use the more technical term end-organ failure.

Some part of the body is the weakest link and *the first symptoms that appear will refer to the functions of this organ,* not to whatever the stressor is. This is why a milk allergy can cause, say, migraines in one person, eczema in another, depression in a third and colitis in a fourth individual.

In Chapter 10 we shall be looking at a whole list of possible target organ symptoms and you will be amazed at the sheer variety of effects.

It has always been one of the major stumbling blocks to acceptance of the widespread allergy, intolerance and maladaptation phenomenon, that symptoms are so unpredictable and do not conform to any recognizable pattern; moreover symptoms shift from day to day, and that always makes doctors suspect hypochondria or imagined symptoms: what are referred to as functional or psychosomatic conditions ("all in the mind").

Now that you are becoming *diet wise* you will understand the nature of the beast, but conventional doctors cannot comfortably think outside the box which defines illness only in terms of recognizable groups of symptoms – so-called syndromes or diseases. It is remarkably weak thinking to me to admit that symptoms A, B and C are legitimate signs of a disease when occurring together, but if they occur randomly these are not to be taken seriously!

If the pioneer group to which I belong did anything majorly constructive it was, more than anything else, to keep hammering home the point that many mysterious symptoms, unknown maladies and highly variable complaints were really one and the same disease: an allergy or intolerance to a food or some other substance. In other words the appearances varied but the underlying cause was quite constant.

9

Brain Allergies

One of the biggest contributions I made in the 80s and 90s was documenting the effects of what may be called "brain allergy." Dwight D. Kalita and William H. Philpott wrote a terrific book on this topic, now sadly out of print, called *Brain Allergies, the Psychonutrient Connection* (Keats, 1991).

The brain is probably the most significant target organ of all. Food-brain reactions can cause a tremendous variety of effects, including but not limited to violent behavior, inappropriate sexual responses, ADD and hyperkinetic syndrome, feeling unreal and depersonalized, hallucination, depression and frank schizophrenia. This is not surprising, since the brain is related to our perceptions and emotions. Any disturbance or malfunction, such as allergic inflammation, might manifest in an infinite variety of ways, since all symptoms are only altered moods and perceptions.

Some public suspicion of this has always been present, as for example in the matter of aphrodisiac properties of foods. I can state categorically that it happens, but I will disappoint my readers by pointing out that no food behaves this way consistently. It's a personal thing. My basic premise throughout this book is that everyone is unique and will react differently to specific foods. Oysters and champagne might work for some. But ice cream and chicken are two that in my experience have provoked powerful and somewhat degrading reactions in the two women concerned.

Robert Burton (1577- 1640), an English cleric in the "City of Dreaming Spires" (Oxford in England), published his famous book *Anatomy of Melancholy* in 1621. In it he said, "Milk, and all that comes of milk, as butter and cheese, curds etc., increase melancholy (whey only excepted, which is most wholesome): some except asses' milk. The rest, to such as are sound, is nutritive and good, especially for young children, but because soon turned to corruption, not good for those that have unclean stomachs, are subject to headache…"

I like his word *corruption* for acquired food intolerance!

Incidentally, I cite this book also as the earliest example of what we now call *journaling*. Burton was prone to melancholy himself and wrote his tract to try and lift himself out of it.

[*Anatomy of Melancholy* is available as a text file from www.gutenberg. net. There are no page numbers but you can use 'search' or 'find' to trace references to milk.]

Brain damage

One of my pioneer causes has been to investigate whether the dietary correction helps people who are brain damaged. It grew out of a teaching from one of my old professors; he said it was wrong to cast aside elderly patients who had symptoms, just because they were old. He pointed out that vitamin supplements might make a big difference; cut the person's toenails; take them for a drive – all these little asides could markedly improve the lot of a senile patient. Just because a major turnaround is no longer possible, it doesn't mean small improvements are not worthwhile! At the very least, they are gestures of compassion.

When I saw the extraordinary recoveries that were possible, using the *diet wise* approach, I remembered his words and asked myself: "We know there is loss of motor or cognitive function but could some performance be recoverable, using the food exclusion principle?

You bet it could.

Casebook 4.

One of the most moving stories of my entire medical career was that of a woman called Susan (her real name). She was thirty-nine years old when she came to me. Her parents had read about me in the newspapers, talking about improvements despite brain damage, and wondered if I could help their daughter in any way.

Susan was indisputably mentally handicapped. She had the mind of a child. She could not read or write; she could not count or deal with money; she was a danger to herself in the kitchen, since she was extremely clumsy and forgetful – the sort of individual who might overlook lighting the gas and blow herself up, or forget that dishes from the oven are very hot and could cause serious burns. Susan couldn't even be allowed to cross the road unaccompanied, for fear of her safety.

But that was all about to change.

Just a few weeks into the *diet wise* plan, exactly as you have it here in these pages, Susan "woke up."

In her own dramatic and moving words, she said, "I just woke up one day and I was here!"

I find it hard to comprehend what that must mean for a woman of almost forty, whose life had been uncomprehending up to that point.

Not that she settled for moping about the lost years.

Susan began learning to read and write; she could count; she could go shopping on her own; she understood money and could obtain the correct change; she wanted to paint and live life to the full.

Her wonderful story was told and retold in the press, most notably by the German-based magazine *Bella,* under the banner "Prisoner No More." The double-page spread began with Susan's remarkable words, which I will quote unaltered:

> *"This morning I tied my own shoelaces – tied them into neat little bows. And I did it all on my own – without any help from Mum or Dad.*
>
> *"You probably think that's no great achievement for a 39-year-old woman but, believe me, it's a very big step and I feel terribly proud.*
>
> *"You see for most of my life I have been classed as "mentally handicapped" and even the simplest tasks were well beyond me.*
>
> *"Although I could see, hear, smell, taste… I simply couldn't understand what my senses were telling me. The messages were all jumbled. So the world passed me by in a confused, bewildering blur.*
>
> *"It's only in the last few months I've come out into the real world – and it's fantastic.*
>
> *"I feel as if I've been reborn or, at least, released from prison after serving a long harsh sentence."*

I could tell even the hard-nosed journalists were really gripped by this drama.

Susan's allergies, when we had discovered them, were beef, dairy products, wheat and tomatoes. Of course she had been fed dairy products from birth and in any case had met all four foods in the womb. Susan was born off-center because of food reactions developed before she even drew her first breath. In her case the target organ was her brain.

Here was a salutary case where over 95% recovery of brain function took place. *Let it be a solemn warning to all, what sad stories may be out there, of people doomed to inadequacy because of unsuspected reactions to humble everyday foods.*

Long afterwards I used to love getting the scrawly letters Susan wrote me. Possibly the deepest moment of all between us was when, on her final visit, she asked if she could work for me and help others in a similar predicament to hers: *"I can answer the phone and write things down!"* she said proudly.

It takes a lot to render me speechless, as friends and family will confirm, but at that moment the lump in my throat was so big I couldn't answer. I just trusted to a hug.

Casebook 5.

A more physically damaged patient was an 18-year-old girl, among my Scottish patients. Angela had cerebral palsy, as a result of severe trauma at birth (forceps, I seem to remember). She had never spoken. She could not move well, due to the stiff spasticity of her limbs. If she slavered and snorted a little, nobody minded: "She's brain damaged. What do you expect?" was what the doctors told her mother.

Then I was called in.

After just ten days on the test diet I have given you in Chapter 11, Angela spoke. Now I do not mean she started to *learn* to speak. She just came out with it. Her very first words (eighteen years of age, remember) were "I love you Mummy!"

Her forbearing mother nearly collapsed with surprise and delight.

What was so moving here was that Angela clearly had understood language all along. Inside she had wanted to be part of everything going on around her and nobody knew she was even at home with the lights on. Too much by far had been taken for granted. Angela must have felt very isolated and dismissed as mentally defective as well as crippled.

You may ask how this recovery was even possible. Well, as I said before, even if there is an incurable problem, there may be some aspect of it that responds to treatment. In this case there was no question that Angela had severe brain damage and spastic limbs; she would never walk unaided. But that did not mean she had zero cognitive function. In fact her brain was probably being as fazed with incompatible food reactions as Susan's. Once that inflammation was settled down, the speech function areas began to recover, along with the frontal lobe areas where we process our feelings.

You would think this story and its outcome was a matter of universal delight. Most newspapers regarded it in that light. But one odious Scottish Sunday newspaper used the story to attack me professionally: "Miracle cure exposed as a fraud" was their headline response. It featured a street shot of me stepping into my Mercedes car, as if that made me some kind of crook preying on the sick and helpless. Years of trouble followed this abusive story. But what sickened me most was their willingness to ignore the true recovery and its implication for others, just to justify their political tirade.

In what sense was the cure a "fraud"? Did Angela pretend to talk? Did her mother fake the reports that her daughter had begun speaking after eighteen years?

Again I am pleased to return to this case because it makes the same point as Susan's: *out there may be many millions of people, imprisoned inside, because food allergy and intolerance is inflaming their brains and preventing proper cognitive function.*

Neurotransmitters

All this was twenty years ago or more. I am relieved that science has somewhat started to move on this.

There are good biochemical reasons why the brain should be especially susceptible to the toxins of allergy reactions. The brain is the only organ in the body that cannot control cell wall permeability. Moreover it seems that food substances can provoke inappropriate levels of on-board morphine-like substances, called endorphins. Food peptides (small proteins) can behave in the same way. These were first reported by Christine Zioudrou, et al. who dubbed such peptides "exorphins." Between the two, food reactions can certainly induce a drug-like haze, inducing a form of stupor, which is seen as fatigue, woolly brain, autism and other learning disabilities. Naturally these "on-site" drug reactions can cause inappropriate stimulation too, leading to aggression, hyperkinetic syndrome and even violence.

Further elucidation of this issue has been provided through the extensive work of Fukudome and Yoshikawa, published over the last decade [Fukudome S, Yoshikawa M. Opioid peptides derived from wheat gluten: their isolation and characterization. FEBS Lett. 1992 Jan 13; 296(1):107-11.] who have identified and characterized five distinct exorphins in the pepsin digests of gluten. Eight distinct exorphins have also been identified in the pepsin digests of milk [Mycroft, FJ, et al. MIF-like sequences in milk and wheat proteins. N Engl. J Med. 1982 Sep 30; 307(14):895].

Frank Dohan has become well known for his contention that exorphins are a major factor in schizophrenia [Dohan, F. C. Genetic hypothesis of idiopathic schizophrenia: its exorphin connection. Schizophr Bull. 1988; 14(4):489-94.]

The field of serology has also provided us with some very clear evidence that such peptides, and the proteins from which they derive, can be absorbed through the intestinal mucosa, and into the circulation of a significant minority of apparently healthy members of the general population [Husby S, Jensenius JC, Svehag SE, Passage of undegraded dietary antigen into the blood of healthy adults. Quantification, estimation of size distribution, and relation of uptake to levels of specific antibodies. Scand J Immunol. 1985 Jul; 22(1):83-92].

Scientists say a minority because they are not measuring many peptides as potential exorphins. They only test for it in wheat and milk and then say studies show it only for wheat and milk. It is easily within the grasp of an average school child that this phenomenon will occur with other peptides too, once they take the trouble to look.

OPIORPHIN

French researchers, under Dr. Catherine Rougeot, from Institut Pasteur in Paris, have identified an endogenous compound, which they have termed Opiorphin, that is comparable to morphine in analgesic potency.

Testing of Opiorphin in the behavioral rat model of acute mechanical pain showed that its analgesic efficacy was on par with that of morphine, the researchers note.

"Our discovery of Opiorphin is extremely exciting from a physiologic point of view in the context of endogenous opioidergic pathways, notably in modulating mood-related states and pain sensation," Dr. Rougeot's team states.

[*Proc Natl Acad Sci* USA 2006;103:17979-17984.]

Intoxication!

The results of brain allergy can be bizarre and hilarious, as well as harrowing.

In 1986 I appeared on a television lunchtime special with Alan Titchmarsh (later of *Ground Force* fame). I was introducing a young girl, Josie, who got drunk eating potatoes.

Really!

Of course the story was so bizarre and entertaining, it was a natural media hit. As I said to Alan, alcohol impairs brain function, at first stimulating it (feeling good), then killing off inhibitions (drunkenness) and finally leading to depression of motor and cognitive function (stupor). It did this simply by selectively poisoning pathways, so that impairment takes place. It's a process familiar to us all (well, most of us!).

Food allergy inflammatory responses can do exactly the same thing, I explained to the viewers. In Josie's case potato was the offender. Alan offered her a plate of fries, which was whipped up from somewhere by the studio backup team, as a joke.

She politely refused.

Josie's mother and father suffered pretty badly with allergies too. We had an interesting discussion and a memorable program, well ahead of its time.

But Josie was far from unique. I had several young women in this predicament. Lynne was sensitive to oranges and got drunk whenever she ate them. The thing was, she didn't know this! All she knew was that when she went drinking with her friends (usually vodka and orange) she became drunk too easily. Thinking alcohol was the problem, she stayed with the orange juice. That had resulted in her dancing on the pub tables. Lynne had always just seemed very excitable and no one had really made the right connections, till she came to me.

The irony in her story was that she was fine on the vodka – it was the orange that made her drunk!

Girls getting silly and out of control on simple foodstuffs could potentially cause them serious problems. Which brings us neatly onto the topic of the next section.

Inappropriate sexual stimulation

There is no question that food reactions can cause an altered sexual response and I want to share this with you.

On the negative side, eating foods that make you sick and dull your senses has a profoundly negative effect on libido and affection. Patients who are affected may shun the touch of another person and turn very nasty when their partner or spouse tries to make physical overtures. I don't think I really need to elaborate on this aspect.

But it will be surprising to most people to know that food can cause inappropriate and even dangerous arousal. Lay folk have a strong belief in the aphrodisiac properties of certain foods, such as champagne, oysters, aniseed and arugula (rocket). Bananas and asparagus have been mentioned too, presumably because of the phallic appearance.

But my work has shown that these reactions are far from universal and mostly illusory. The Scott-Mumby truth is that any food can act as an aphrodisiac, if it provokes the right reaction in the brain. This is simply a different target organ phenomenon; some people get headaches, some joint pains – some become aroused! It's not common but does occur.

You may find this happens to you, when we come to the food challenge tests in Chapter 12.

One of my patients carried out an eating challenge with strong coffee. She was surprised to be quite turned on; so much so she masturbated and then felt ashamed and wanted to shower afterwards. Another woman in her 50s ate ice cream for the first time after months on a dairy-free regime and was so aroused that she grabbed a hapless youth and took him to bed for wild sex. The boy probably didn't know what hit him – but I knew what had hit her and she was mighty relieved when I explained it to her. I am concerned that on some occasions this must happen to people, who find themselves in difficult situations as a result, without having the least idea why they were suddenly provoked to such unaccustomed behavior.

The UPs and DOWNs of addiction

Theron "Ted" Randolph MD, the late doyen of the allergy and ecology movement, produced a wonderful insightful table, showing the effects of alternate stimulation and suppression of brain and mind function, caused by food and drink triggers. Over twenty years ago he gave me permission to quote it widely and I have worked to popularize it since.

It is important to remember that stimulation and suppression can take place simultaneously as well as longitudinally. We all know that alcohol, for instance, will stimulate and then later suppress (drunk then stuporose). But if you grasp that it makes a person drunk by suppressing inhibitions, then this will make more sense.

Stimulatory and Withdrawal Levels and Manifestations

+4	manic, with or without convusions	distraught, excited, agitated, enraged and panicky; circuitous or one-track thoughts, muscle twitching and jerking of extremities, convulsive siezures and altered consciousness may develop.
+3	hypomanic, toxic, anxious and egocentric	aggressive, loquacious, clumsy (ataxic), anxious, fearful and apprehensive, alternating chills and flushing, ravenous hunger, excessive thirst; giggling or pathological laughter may occur.
+2	hyperactive, irritable, hungry and thirsty	tense, jittery, hopped up, talkative, argumentative, sensitive, overly responsive, self-centered, hungry and thirsty; flushing, sweating and chilling may occur, as well as insomnia, alcoholism and obesity.
+1	stimulated but relatively symptom free	active, alert, lively, responsive and enthusiastic, with unimpaired ambition, energy, initiative and wit; considerate of the views and actions of others; this usually comes to be regarded as "normal" behavior.
0	behavior on an even keel, as in homeostasis	children expect this from their parents and teachers, parents expect this from their children, we all expect it from our associates.
-1	localized allergic manifestations	running or stuffy nose, clearing throat, coughing, wheezing, itching, eczema and hives, gas, diarrhea, constipation, colitic, urgency and frequency of urination, various eye and ear syndromes.
-2	systemic allergic reactions	tired, dopey, somnolent, mildly depressed, odematous, with painful syndromes (headache, neckache, backache, neuralgia, myalgia, myositis, arthralgia, arthritis, arteritis, chest pain) and cardiovascular effects
-3	depressions and distrurbed mentation	confused, indecisive, moody, sad, sullen, withdrawn or apathetic; emotional instablity and impaired attention, concentration, comprehension and thought processes (loss of speech, mental lapses and blackouts)
-4	severe depression, with or without lowered consciousness	non-responsive, lethargic, stuporose, disoriented, melancholic, incontinent, regressive thinking, paranoid orientations, delusions, hallucinations, sometimes amnesia and finally comatose

Violence

The fact is that allergies and intolerance to foods can produce inappropriate stimulation, as well as depression of function. Not surprisingly therefore, violence was one of the problems I frequently had to investigate and try to solve. That could be a child suffering "smashing up" attacks or an adult disposed to murderous violence, after eating trigger foods.

It is notorious in the police force that Christmas is a time of peak family violence. I'm speaking here about Britain, where we don't have a Thanksgiving equivalent, but I did notice a 2005 news item, reporting that four 17-year-olds were killed in Boston over Thanksgiving and a quadruple homicide claimed four more young people in a Dorchester basement.

This might seem paradoxical in the season of good will; but I have a possible explanation, based on what I've observed over the years. What do we all do most of in the festive season? Eat and drink! In fact our intake over that period is so excessive that the majority of people, if they are honest, feel rather below par. Just too much spuds, stuffing, pudding, cakes and ale wreak havoc on our bodies and minds. For most people that means feeling depressed and wanting to sleep on the sofa. But the reader will now surely recognize that for some people, that means disturbed brain function, hyperstimulation and inappropriate emotions, all waiting to come out as aggression. No studies have ever been done on this but I feel my hypothesis is a very strong one. If your family is prone to rows at Christmas or Thanksgiving, consider this a possibility and get smart about it.

Super-strength child

Probably my most outstanding case of child rages was David, a young boy of five from Ireland, whose outbursts were so extreme that parents truly did have to nail down the furniture. Incredible though it seems for a child of that age, he was able to muster enough strength to tear a door from its hinges. His distraught parents explained that they *really did* have to nail down the furniture. His allergy turned out to be wheat, mainly. His parents had figured that out by following the instructions given in my first edition of this book, *The Food Allergy Plan,* and when we finally got together in Manchester I was able to confirm their findings and add some new aspects to origins of the problem.

Ultimately, David, his mother and I went together on Gay Byrne's show. Almost every soul in Ireland listened in to Gay, who was the Irish equivalent of Larry King! I wanted to say that David's whole problem had started as a result of his measles vaccination; he was fine up to that point and then deteriorated very badly. This caused pandemonium in the studio and eventually I had to settle for saying "it seems as if…" Gay was very insistent on this point.

As a result of appearing on the hugely popular show, the telephone exploded and I had so many calls from distraught parents asking if I could help their child, that I took it as a call to open a third clinic in Dublin. I had happy times there and enjoyed plenty of the *craic* (Gaelic for fun and camaraderie).

Attempted murder

At the other end of the scale was an older youth, also Irish, called Tony. In 1987 he was referred to me by the British Courts for an evaluation. Tony had been charged with attempted murder, later mitigated to grievous bodily harm, after trying to strangle his stepfather. This forbearing man had heard of my work with violent youths and asked the judge to consider this might be the reason for his stepson's violent outbursts. His request was granted and Tony was sent to my office. He was not under guard.

Because of the exigencies and imperatives of the situation, I decided to use intradermal challenge testing. This required injecting tiny amounts of food extract. All the more remarkable therefore that some of the reactions we observed were severe. On two occasions I was called to deal with Tony's threatening outbursts, which terrified my nurses. But each reaction was quite clear and the corresponding "neutralizing dose" quelled his rage, proving equally reliably that the effect was a reaction to specific foods.

In fact potato, beef, strawberry and one other food I have since forgotten had this effect on him – but no other common food. The worst reaction was to potato, and pretty soon the media, who were already watching the case because of the court connection, launched into a frenzy of irony that an Irish youth should be allergic to potato. Tony became known as the "Irish Potato Boy" and his story reverberated round the world. I had an unheard-of forty-minute news slot on prime time TV (Channel 4 UK) and the production team came to film me at work. Tony certainly obliged with a reaction in front of the camera, sweating, shaking and looking murderous, right on cue after an injection.

In due course Tony was found guilty and given a conditional discharge, the condition being that he stick to my diet regime and stay out of trouble. Months later I heard that the judge himself had watched the

Channel 4 newscast. My hat is off to him as an enlightened and intelligent man. I made medico-legal history: this was the first time that food allergy was accepted by a court as a provocation factor in violence.

Epilepsy

One of the conditions with which I scored an early success was the treatment of epilepsy. It was never suggested at medical school that this condition could be modified or eliminated, except by miraculous grace.

In fact I found that incompatible foods were common triggers and had some remarkable recoveries over the years. One man was intolerant of wheat and that brought on fits; as soon as we discovered this, he gave up eating wheat and never had another attack. We even managed to get back his driving license, the authorities were so impressed with my evidence.

Another outstanding case was a boy of eleven, who reacted to carrot and related foods. You will learn later about food families (Chapter 15); in this case the foods related to carrot are parsley, parsnip, celery, dill, fennel and coriander (cilantro). The young lad himself noticed they all have the same frilly green tops! In his case the whole food family was bad news – if he ate even small traces of them he began having seizures. But, once again, he was fine off the foods and did not require Epanutin for maintenance. This was fortunate, given the long-term ill effects of that class of drugs.

I longed to do studies with an EEG machine but could find no help from the local hospitals. However there have been clues, published over the decades, that food can upset brain electrical activity: a study geared towards depression, rather than epilepsy, showed abnormal electrical activity in more than two thirds of untreated children returned to normal foods, following dietary restriction such as I have described repeatedly in these pages. [Paul K, Todt J, Eysold R. EEG Research Findings in Children with Celiac Disease According to Dietary Variations. Zeitschrift der Klinische Medizin 1985; 40: 707-709; Corvaglia L, et al. Depression in adult untreated celiac subjects: diagnosis by the pediatrician. Am J Gastroenterol. 1999 Mar; 94(3):839-43]

Incidentally, orthodox medicine is now catching up with my clinical discoveries. I noticed recently a paper in which certain types of epilepsy are now recognized in association with celiac disease. Celiac disease is, of course, understood to be due primarily to a gluten allergy [Gobbi et al. (1992) The Lancet 340:439-443]

Miscellaneous neurological conditions improve

Beyond purely brain allergy, certain conditions of the nerves and muscles are also worth investigating with my diet technique. You have probably heard that multiple sclerosis (MS) can be aggravated by food and other allergies. In those early years there were few of us working on that problem but the results were sometimes impressive. I have had cases get up from wheelchairs and at times it seemed like a miracle. In fact it was so hard to believe that we probably attracted a lot of unnecessary hostility from colleagues by even attempting to improve this condition.

But the logic is simple. If nerve tissue is inflamed and non-functional but not dead, then it may recover useful function. One of the commonest provocations of inflammation is allergies and therefore unburdening allergies, especially foods, was likely to be beneficial. The inflammation dies down, the nerves work once more and the patient regains the ability to walk normally. Heavy metal toxicity is another potent cause of provocation, incidentally.

The settling of the inflammation model would also probably suffice to explain other neurological recoveries, from ALS and motor neurone disease, or Parkinsonism and Alzheimer's. I've helped them all, many times, but I could never get a clear marker for who would respond and who wouldn't. If you or a loved one has one of these conditions, I can only say it is worth giving the diet a try. As I used to reason with patients, even if science eventually proved it could help only one in a hundred cases, you would be very happy if you were that hundredth person!

Muscular dystrophy

Finally in this section, I'd like to share another of my miracle cases that left me in awe and with a wonderful sense of being blessed and helped by higher forces. It concerns a young 6-year-old boy called Ryan, with muscular dystrophy. This is a progressive condition of muscular weakness and wasting, which starts in the legs and pelvis and later affects the whole body, usually resulting in early death due to respiratory or heart failure. It is a genetic disorder, either inherited or caused by a gene mutation, and affects males almost exclusively.

There is no question Ryan had this disorder. It shows up before the 6th year of life and the first thing that parents notice, usually, is the child using his arms and hands to push himself upright, instead of leg muscles.

His parents brought Ryan to see me to ask if I could help. These were heady pioneer days and my frequent appearances in the press and on TV and radio, featuring some surprising recoveries, allowed many intelligent parents to reasonably question whether a prognosis of "incurable" was really correct. Given the gloomy outlook for Ryan, I was willing to try.

Looking back, I was being remarkably cocky, maybe even arrogant, but in fact it wasn't even difficult. Within two weeks on the program in this book Ryan was on the road to recovery. The first exciting report was that his parents saw Ryan running alongside a friend on his bicycle. That didn't sound like progressive muscular weakness! In fact he made such a good recovery that one day not long afterwards Ryan climbed the Walter Scott Monument in Edinburgh, Scotland. The structure is 200 feet high and has 287 steps. There is an official certificate for those who climb to the top and Ryan was the proud possessor of one.

At the time, even I had to admit it shouldn't have happened. But I did recognize this is the power of the body load model. If you reduce the body's burden by whatever means, then partial or complete recovery is likely to take place. Diet is the most dramatic unburdening route I know, and relatively easy to do, once you have absorbed the contents of this book. Being truly diet wise is very powerful and can help you with so many health issues in life.

A quarter of a century on, I would now think in terms of genetic food programming. Genes and minor gene variants called SNPs (single nucleotide polymorphs) mean that we are all virtually unique in our responses to food. But as I have hinted earlier, we now know that gene expression in turn can be influenced by environmental exposures to many substances, including what we eat. Almost certainly in this case I was able to down-regulate Ryan's dystrophic gene and so put his lethal illness into reverse.

To generalize from this exciting new theory of gene control, it means if you find and follow your own personalized diet, as I explain in these pages, then you are in fine shape to live far longer and conquer major killers, such as cancer and heart disease. Your good genes will flourish and your bad genes will regress. At last I'm sure you are beginning to understand why Luigi Cornaro (page 6) lived against all odds to reach the age of ninety-eight years, at a time when few survived their fortieth birthday and when it was quite exceptional even to reach the Biblical three score years and ten. Cornaro not only lived a long time but was remarkably fit and well, providing he remained *diet wise*!

Now it is time to take stock of your own health status and get started on changing it for the better. What follows in the next chapter is a survey of symptoms, arranged by target organ...

10

Self Inventory

First of all, let's find out where you are starting from: what is your present state of health, really? A lot of people are inclined to minimize symptoms and shrug them off. Perhaps this is due to a fear of admitting something is wrong; or simply to the fact that the body adapts so wonderfully, compensating for defects, that the illness steals up on it unnoticed. The latter would explain why some patients only report to the doctor when they are critically ill and disease has progressed much too far.

Just remember, a symptom, no matter how slight, is the body's way of crying out 'Help!' A symptom, in a way, is a helpful friendly sign that is trying to tell you something. But you must pay attention and make changes, otherwise the problem moves to the next stage, which is a serious breakdown.

Five key symptoms

Dr Richard Mackarness gave five key symptoms that point the way to allergic illness and that have special importance. He believed that without one of the following symptoms, diagnosis is unlikely:

1. Over- or under-weight or fluctuating weight
2 Persistent fatigue that isn't helped by rest.
3. Occasional swellings around the eyes, hands, abdomen, ankles, etc.
4. Palpitations or speeded heart rate, particularly after meals
5. Excessive sweating, not related to exercise

It needs mentioning that there should be no other explanation for these symptoms.

Many people experience symptoms that are quite indicative of an allergy or intolerance, without realizing it. Patients sometimes say that peeling potatoes makes their hands sting; but it never occurred to them that swallowing the vegetable might do internal harm.

Some people are sensitive to lemon and limes and get brown itchy patches on the skin of the hands after handling these fruits. It is usually made worse by exposure to sunlight. Eating figs and celery can produce the photosensitizing effect too.

In fact we can use skin inflammation as a test for allergies, when someone is too ill or too tiny to cooperate (as with a small baby). If you slice a food and apply the raw surface to the skin for just a few minutes, you can often see a significant reddening, which would indicate it is an irritant and therefore should not be swallowed.

This works especially well with fruits.

If you are aware of *any* reaction to a food that is out of the ordinary, be sure to include it in the self-inventory.

The number one question

Over the years, I learned that one magic question, more than all the others I will share with you in this chapter, gave the strongest pointer to allergy and intolerance.

Do your symptoms come and go frequently?

Healthy one day, ill the next, then well again a couple of days later is a huge waving banner, which gives away the whole story to an alert physician!

An allergy or intolerance reaction, to food or to other substances, is almost the only pathological mechanism which will give rise to this quickly shifting pattern. Think about it. Infection with micro-organisms will not come and go in this manner: if you have an infection it will take at least a week or more to clear, however brilliant your immune system. Parasites and certain stealth viruses may not declare themselves at all but are certainly not going to appear and disappear within the body over a matter of hours or days. Degenerative diseases progress steadily: if you have diabetes, arthritis, arteriosclerosis or other cardiovascular damage, macular degeneration of the retina, diverticulitis or senescent skin, then you will experience long slow changes with very little relapse (unless you follow the advice in this book!). Tumors (malignant or benign) enlarge steadily and do not shrink one day and re-appear the next.

No; sudden inflammation, due to an allergy or intolerance is about the only disease process which has this characteristic abrupt and intermittent behavior. The body is basically sound but something is attacking it on a frequent basis – often daily, as we shall see.

The corollary to this number-one question, incidentally, gives rise to one of my most valuable sayings and one which inspired patients the most: *if you can be symptom-free on any day you can be symptom free every day.* It's obvious. If even just one day a year all symptoms clear up and you feel fine, then there is nothing structurally wrong, nothing missing, no broken parts, no fatal flaw in your body's defenses. In the classic phrase: there is a healthy you inside, just waiting to get out! You're really fine.

But, of course, you need to know what it is that is knocking you off healthy and well. That's the culprit I'm calling an allergy or intolerance. The chances are it (or they) is a toxic food.

Organ by organ

Let's look for more clues. We'll consider symptoms organ by organ, or system by system. In general, you should concentrate on the last twelve months, if you have been continuously ill in that period. You may then take a wider view and consider which symptoms have been present, on and off, *since you became ill.*

Eyes

Do you have red, itchy eyes, a gritty feeling in the eyes, that makes your eyes water? Do you have dark rings under the eye? (We call these "allergic shiners" because they can look just like a bruised or "black eye"). Do your eyes have an unnatural 'sparkle'? In children especially, that is a sign I see often. Blurring of vision, spots in view, flashing lights and double vision are four symptoms that may be transient and caused by allergy and intolerance.

However there may be a more serious explanation for this quartet and you should consult a physician before dismissing them as diet related.

Classic "floaters" (dark flecks circulating within your field of view) I have noticed can be caused or made worse by allergic reactions.

Skin

The surface of your body is a classic marker for signs an allergy. Probably the most outstanding allergy rash we call urticaria; it is hot, itchy and raised in bumps, like a nettle sting (*Urtica* is the Latin word for nettle). A variant of that, called giant urticaria, is really about fluids escaping from the blood vessels, causing major swellings. This can be so bad as to close a person's throat and cause difficulty breathing. Arguably, it is but a short step from this to anaphylaxis, the dread and often fatal allergic reaction, in which the patient passes rapidly into shock and circulatory collapse.

Another interesting variant we call *dermographia*, which literally means "skin writing." When the skin is this sensitive, slight pressure on the skin produces the typical urticarial wheal. Just stroking the skin of the back would make it possible to write words, which emerge as wheals – hence the name of this condition. But the same effect occurs where buckles, bra straps, elastic knickers and other pressure points irritate the skin.

Eczema is a common and debilitating skin eruption that can make life miserable due to itching and scratching. Often it goes with asthma and hay fever in a combination we call "atopic", meaning an inherited severe generalized allergy tendency. Such individuals are often in a miserable condition, hardly able to live normally; they look bright red (inflammation), scratch and wheeze, and may deposit skin flakes on the rug and in bed like a biological snow. Stress seems to play a part too, exacerbating the condition relentlessly.

Atopy is tougher but still responds extremely well to discovering and following the right diet, which reduces the system overload and allows recovery.

Casebook 6.

This is a good point to relate the case in which an infant literally peed himself back to size! At the age of eight months he had severe eczema – so bad in fact that physicians had even tried steroid creams, in desperation (a very serious and dangerous undertaking in one so young and with this condition, because of the quantity of steroid drug absorbed through the skin). Even this drastic measure had failed and the child had been sent home, more or less with the intimation he would probably die.

The parents were desperate and brought him to me. The baby was a sorry mess, swollen, red and wheezing, with skin that was over 90% cracked, weeping and bloody in places. When his diaper came off, sheets of skin adhered to it.

I began with a diet survey exactly as you will be asked to do later in this chapter. In a few minutes I had the answer! Potato was the only food that came up over and over on a daily basis – I have already explained how significant that is. Moreover I have found over the years that potato comes up unusually frequently as a cause of eczema – a tip worth remembering if you have this skin condition.

I told the parents to take potato out of the kiddie's diet, compiled a whole range of alternative foods and rotated everything he was eating (see Chapter 15 for details of rotation dieting).

Two days later they called me, very excited. Already the child's skin lesions had closed in most places. But most strikingly, he had peed and peed, soaking dozens of diapers, and literally shrunk to size before their eyes. His bloating had been a reaction to the allergy, just as swollen fingers and eyes often are.

Despite the drama of the success, the parents told me later they hadn't quite believed my explanation and had given the child fries, to see what would happen. That night he had erupted in itching and had torn at his skin until it bled.

They were convinced.

Ear, throat, nose and mouth

Symptoms in this zone are often ignored or made light of by regular physicians. However, many vague or subjective symptoms can be provoked by food allergy and intolerance and, conversely, will disappear when the allergy is addressed – causing immense relief.

Catarrh, post-nasal drip, feeling bunged up, sneezing and runny nose are probably the most characteristic symptoms. We lump these together as *rhinitis* (literally Greek "nose inflammation"). Seasonal rhinitis usually refers to hay fever or summer catarrh. However I have written that seasonal may mean in winter, when we go indoors and shut ourselves in with the furnace fumes and house dust!

Perennial rhinitis refers to all-year-round catarrh and usually means a food – but don't forget, some foods are seasonal. Milk is famous for "thickening the catarrh." That's how common this problem is.

Less commonly I have encountered a metallic taste, mouth (aphthous) ulcers and stiffness of throat or tongue.

In children, the outstanding identifier of food reactions is repeated sore throats and ear infections. Time and again this responds to simple measures, such as a dairy-free diet. Sadly, doctors tend to use antibiotics over and over, sometimes several times a year, without ever questioning there was some cause beyond a bug or virus. The tragedy is that such overuse of antibiotics will often lead to yeast and mold infections in the gut, further reinforcing the dietary overload mechanism.

Cardiovascular system

Care is needed here, because there can be, of course, serious processes underlying cardiovascular dysfunction. For decades I have known that food allergy and intolerance is *the* major cause of hypertension, not supposed arteriosclerosis. How do I discriminate? Easy. If ever, on any occasion, the patient has a reasonable blood pressure, even just one reading in twenty, *hardening of the arteries cannot be the problem*. Doctors miss this vital point.

A week or two on the Stone Age elimination program is enough to bring blood pressure back to normal 95% of the time. Reversing the exclusions, by reintroducing the foods one at a time and seeing which food is the culprit that raises blood pressure is simple and satisfying to do. Patients feel really empowered and "in charge" of the situation, without relying on drugs.

We shall see later that speeded (resting) pulse after food is such a clear sign of an allergic or intolerant reaction that I actually suggest measuring it as part of formal testing. If you get palpitations, especially after eating, don't panic. It's almost certainly a sign of allergy or intolerance; any food can do it, not just caffeine.

Lungs

The lungs are very sensitive barometers of body stress, as asthma suffers will attest. Yet doctors persistently miss addressing the possibility that food will affect the lungs, being blindly intent that only inhaled allergens can cause a problem. Wheezing, tightness and poor respiratory function are key signs of allergic bronchospasm.

Beware the cough – many asthma cases begin as a cough and are misdiagnosed, sometimes for years, as "bronchitis." The latter is essentially an infective disease and believing it to be the diagnosis, doctor may prescribe antibiotics quite inappropriately.

Gastro-intestinal

Symptoms of food allergy or genetic food intolerance are almost certain to disturb the alimentary tract. Symptoms related to this target organ can thus be many and varied and will include nausea, vomiting, belching, 'stomach rumbling,' hunger pangs, "acidity," dyspepsia (indigestion, not all the time), abdominal bloating, flatulence, diarrhea, constipation and variability of bowel function (switching one to the other).

I tackled many peptic ulcers as potential food allergy and got some surprisingly good results. We now know that an organism called *Helicobacteria pylori* is involved. Of course doctors have quickly and illogically jumped to the conclusion that this is the "cause" of peptic ulceration. There is now a supposed proper treatment, which is the much abused antibiotic. Try dietary changes first and see if that does not eliminate the "cause" just as easily.

Musculo-skeletal complaints

Symptoms in this system can include swollen and painful joints, aching muscles, stiffness, cramps, what the British call 'Fibrositis,' another that the world over calls "rheumatism" (temperature-sensitive aches and pains), muscle spasms, tremors (shaking, especially on waking) and pseudo-paralysis.

Genito-urinary system

Several linked symptoms here: menstrual difficulties (so-called endometriosis often responds very well), frequency of urination, bed-wetting (especially in later years), burning urination, genital itch and urgency.

Significant urinary and menstrual disturbance should always be investigated by the conventional route, before opting for a holistic approach.

Resumption of menstrual bleeding after the menopause should always be regarded with deep suspicion.

Headache

The head is not an organ, as such. But there are many varieties of headache encountered, including the following:

Migraine
'Sick headaches': Pressure, Throbbing, Stabbing
'Solid' feeling
Mild or moderate headaches
Stiff neck

Nervous system and mental state

I have already alluded to the complex and infinitely diverse nature of reactions from the brain and nervous system. Nevertheless, to help you, I have singled out the following symptoms that you may recognize:

Inability to think clearly
'Dopey' feeling
Terrible thoughts on waking
Insomnia
Crabby on waking
Difficulty waking up
Bad dreams
Light headedness
Twitching
Memory loss
Stammering
Math and spelling errors
'Blankness'
Delusion
Hallucination
Desire to injure oneself
Convulsions
Stimulated, excited, giddy, silly
Intoxication
Hyperactivity

Tension
Restlessness
Fidgeting
Restless legs
Anxiety
Panic attacks
Irritability
Uncontrollable rage
Smashing-up attacks
General speeding-up
Depressed
'Brain fog' or "wooly brain syndrome"
Withdrawn
Melancholy
Confused
Crying
Lack of confidence
Unreal
Depersonalized
Low mood

The following symptoms are hard to classify, but definitely revealing:

Falling asleep after eating
Sudden chills after eating
Eating binges
Any abrupt change of state from well to unwell
Feeling totally drained and exhausted
Flu-like state that isn't flu
Feeling unwell all over

There can be other reasons for these symptoms – none of them are exclusive to food reactions. But in my experience, the more of these symptoms you suffer from the more certain it is that you have a food allergy or intolerance; in other words: you are reacting to a toxic food.

Quite a list – and probably far from complete. Patients come up with new variations all the time. If you don't recognize or understand an item from the table, don't worry: the chances are that if it means nothing to you then you don't experience it.

Flatulence

Flatulence is a Latin word which simply means "blowing off" (Latin: *flatus,* a blowing). The commoner European slang, farting, comes from Old High German, *Ferzen,* which certainly influenced the English language, via the Saxons. The embarrassment, of course, is not really in the word but in the smell (though in our family we had a tradition that the silent events were the smelliest, sbd = "silent but deadly").

On a direct par with bloating, flatulence is one of the major recurring symptoms of which food allergics complain. Bloating is caused by gas in the intestine, mainly the colon. If the gas becomes excessive, flatulence results. It can come and go very dramatically. I have seen patients during a food challenge test enlarge in a matter of one or two minutes, putting on as much as 8 in/20 cm.

There is no comprehensive physiological explanation as to where the gas comes from or, if not expelled via the anus, where it goes. Perhaps it is reabsorbed – but this seems a bit unlikely in view of the obvious volume involved. One of medicine's great mysteries, but not one likely to attract a would-be Nobel prize-winner!

The fact is, any allergy can cause flatulence but certain groups of foods are particularly associated with it: the pulses are notorious, beans and wind often being the subject of crude jokes; brassicas (cabbage, cauliflower, kale etc.) are not as widely recognized but are just as much trouble. Remember, it is not necessarily every member of a food family that causes a reaction.

Lastly, the yeast syndrome, dysbiosis or intestinal fermentation syndrome (Chapter 21), causes much flatulence.

Interesting groups of symptoms

Bloating, pains, palpitations, sudden tiredness, indeed any symptom experienced *shortly after food*, is likely, though not certain, to have food as its cause. Moreover, if your illness is accompanied by gastro-intestinal disturbances, such as pains, flatulence, nausea, and so on, food is very likely to be the culprit, whatever the complaint.

Another whole group of symptoms that are often ignored or glossed over are the mental manifestations. Because few doctors know what they are dealing with they tend to dismiss important clues like these as merely signs of a neurotic personality. Yet tiredness, irritability and low mood are not *normal,* no matter how common. It is a pity so many people accept this unquestioningly as their lot in life. A poor marriage, a stressful job or financial worries are often assigned to the cause of feeling unwell, and it is true that these factors can aggravate symptoms; but as anyone who has been through the *diet wise* plan will tell you, the mere avoidance of the most harmful foods leads to a startling increase in verve, alertness, enthusiasm and willingness to cope with life's setbacks. Stress then becomes secondary: it is easy to conquer if you are feeling terrific!

A lot of us live in a kind of mental 'fog' without recognizing its existence. This is easy to understand, since for many *it never lifts!* But if you have ever had flashes, albeit briefly, of feeling young again and that the world sparkles with joy, as it did when you were a child, then that is *what you are really like*. Think about it.

Saddest of all is that many young children are compelled to grow up facing this unseen barrier to learning and maturing. I'm talking about ADD or ADHD and naughty behavior. Lack of concentration and forgetfulness at school can have disastrous consequences for the rest of a person's life, yet it is one of the commonest of allergy and intolerance symptoms. I often see children who are struggling with emotional burdens and having great difficulties with school studies. Their diets are dreadful, but no one has suggested the real cause of the problem. Time and again the plan has sorted out their dietary liabilities and they have gone on to do very well academically, which proves to me that allergies have this markedly negative effect.

Casebook 7. Maxine's story

One of my early patients was a young girl whom I shall call Maxine. Her case was seized upon by the media, and she became an overnight 'star' with her name in several national newspapers. When I first interviewed her and her parents, Maxine was moody, truculent and unhappy: Her school work placed her at resounding class bottom; she had few friends; she vexed her parents; but, worst of all, her teachers made no secret of their dislike for her. Finally, as if that were not enough, she suffered from terrible migraine. Things had reached crisis point when it was suggested by the head of the school that Maxine's parents should take her to a child psychiatrist. Like many of us they had a suspicious dislike of doctors of that persuasion, but being sensible people and teachers themselves they did realize that something would have to be done. Luckily, about that time they heard about my clinic in Stockport, already internationally known, and decided to come and see me.

To cut a long story short, we found Maxine to be allergic to a wide variety of foods, including wheat, corn, egg, tea, beef, pork and yeast. Her reaction to onion was interesting. Temper tantrums were apparently a feature of Sunday evenings, and bearing in mind the above history it is easy to understand that the parents had naturally ascribed these to a resistance to going to school next day. However, it turned out that weekly Sunday roast *and onions* was the real culprit! Since that time I'm told that Maxine hasn't had a single headache, but the truly remarkable aspect of her recovery is the way her schoolwork has improved beyond all recognition. She moved to the top of the class in some subjects and came very near it in several others. Lo and behold, as a student she was not dim and uncomprehending but actually very bright!

Judging by her relationships with others, Maxine became a new person, garrulous and extrovert, making friends easily. She began to bring friends home and no longer frightened them off with her wild behavior. Teachers recognized the improvement, and this time a letter from the head of the school, instead of complaining, was full of pleasant surprise and inquired what might be the cause of the change.

The flood of calls and letters we received after Maxine's story was publicized revealed that, all too sadly, her case was far from unique. A great many anxious parents whose children have similar problems are at their wits' end, wondering what to do. The tragedy of it is that the steps needed are so very simple: a few days on the diet given in the next chapter is all it would take for most of such children to recover and begin to behave normally; for the rest, advice given later in the book would provide a remedy.

The effect of poor eating on our future generations is quite devastating. The harm it does tends to be self-perpetuating. *All* parents should study this book and its implications; teachers too.

A later chapter looks at the special problems associated with children's food reactions.

How often do you eat the suspect food?

Now we come to look at your own diet. What exactly are you eating?

The key question in this is *how often* do you eat the food, not *how much*. Start by making a list of foods you eat every single day. You'll be surprised how repetitive our daily foods are. Most people will admit to tea or coffee, or both, every day. But does that include milk? Sugar?

What about bread? Another common daily food. Breakfast corn cereal maybe. That would mean milk too and probably sugar (most cereals have the sugar already added. Corn flakes, for example, are about two-thirds sugar by weight. Potato is another food to watch out for; it occurs as fries, mashed potatoes, crusts and chips.

Then go on to make a list of frequently eaten foods. For the purposes of this inventory that means *twice a week or more*. It takes food about four days to clear from the bowel, so if you eat a substance twice weekly it is permanently inside you and could be making you ill without you knowing.

Ignore seasonal variations or foods that you are only temporarily eating more of *unless* this coincides with a period of increased symptoms.

You have developed quite a list of possible suspects. You probably understand by now that your troubles may be coming from a hidden allergy food which is already on this list. Notice how certain food ingredients come up repetitively. Wheat, for instance, appears in bread, cakes, cookies, muffins, pastry, pizza, pasta and other places. Appendix B contains a list of frequent food contacts that you can review. You'll probably be amazed how often some of these turn up but it will be apparent that the chief danger comes from manufactured foods, where you cannot be sure what is included in the can or package, without reading the list of ingredients. Whole food eating has many advantages, one of which is being able to see and identify what you are putting in your mouth!

Two more lists

Now, to complete this inventory make two more lists. These are personal to you. First, a list of foods you know disagree with you. Do not include things you may have been *told* are bad for you (for example, you may have heard that chocolate is bad for migraines); include only those which you have found out *by actual experience* make you ill when you eat them. Secondly, a list of foods you crave or would binge on if you let yourself. If that doesn't have any meaning for you, then try to think of it as a list of things you couldn't give up easily.

The first list may be quite revealing. It is amazing how many people already know that foods can make them ill and yet never realize that their diseases are so caused also. Sometimes a patient will inform me that he or she cannot eat pork because it causes unpleasant symptoms, yet he or she has bacon for breakfast almost daily! Similar cases are milk and beef or chicken and egg (each pair comes from the same animal).

The second list contains clues to likely addictions. However, these are not necessarily the foods that are making you ill. Tea, coffee and chocolate are highly addictive substances. I try to get patients to think of them as drugs because they have true pharmacological actions on the heart, kidneys and brain. Chocolate can on occasion make people very ill and is one of the well-known triggers of migraine, *but unless you eat it regularly, more than once a week, it is not what we are looking for.* Nevertheless, put these binge foods down. Make no mistake, they can cause symptoms.

How good are you on your BEST day?

Finally, we get to look at something cheerful. This is really a crucial self-inventory question that you should ask yourself. How do you feel on your best days? Do you actually have spells when you are completely free of symptoms?

This is important if you do because, as I explain to patients, you can always be at least as good as you are on your best days. It's another Scott-Mumby maxim that if you can feel good for one day, you can feel good every day. Follow the logic: if you can be pretty well sometimes it means there is no serious defect in your body, nothing is broken that can't be fixed. Doctors will tell you that you will experience pain every day from arthritis. But what if some days the pain isn't there? Doesn't that ruin the explanation that the pain comes from the arthritis? Pain may come and go from day to day but joint damage does not.

I recall a case of a man in his fifties, let's call him James, who lived a pretty poor lifestyle and had a serious limp, due to severe arthritis of the hip. He was scheduled soon for a hip replacement. I persuaded him to try the plan described in this book and grudgingly he did so. He was very surprised that by the end of the first week the pain and limp had gone. Unfortunately, after only three weeks of relief he reverted to his old habits.

This is a very instructive story because James could not cope with continuous attention to diet and so gave in to the pressures to have the hip replacement. He described the head of the femur as looking like a mass of accumulated candle wax (the operation was done under local anesthetic and he got to see inside his own hip joint).

James argued that what was found at operation proved that the hip joint was finished and my notions of a cure were absurd. I tried to get him to see that even with a hip so deformed he had been completely pain free and that Nature could have done the repair, given time. He was never convinced.

James died a few years later of a stroke, a common exit for people who take too much cocaine.

Just remember his story: if your symptoms go away, even for just one day, you can be without them for life!

Review the lists

Now is the time to look over the above lists objectively. Ask yourself, what looks unnatural? Potato chips are an occasional indulgence for most of us. But one of my patients consumed five bags of them *every day,* along with, incidentally, two chocolate bars. She had already had one nervous breakdown and was rapidly heading for another, despite heavy doses of tranquillizers. Not surprisingly, these excesses turned out to be contributing to her illness. But the point I am trying to make is that you only had to *look* at her diet to realize it was abnormal:

Five slices of bread a day, ten cups of coffee, two or three bananas – these are all suspicious amounts when judged objectively. Does your list reveal similar flaws? Be honest and underline foods that you are overdoing; cut them out as part of the elimination diet in the next chapter *whether specifically banned or not.*

That completes the inventory, then. Somewhere staring you in the face on these lists may be one or more foods that have been making you suffer unnecessarily for years. Keep these records: there may be valuable information buried in them, for use later on. Also, you may use the list of symptoms as an objective guide to what progress you are making. Sometimes patients feel so well they begin to forget what terrible symptoms they started out with!

The question remains: do you have toxic foods? The only way to find out is to follow the next step in the *Diet Wise* plan.

First, a brief note for cancer sufferers...

Cancer Diets

The individualistic diet approach outlined in this book, I found to be enormously helpful to cancer sufferers. Over the years, my patients (many of whom had cancer, whether they came to see me for that reason or not), did incredibly well and did not experience a recurrence.

I can only speculate that this was due to reducing the immune burden, by getting rid of toxic and allergic foods. As you probably know, cancer is best seen as a disease of the immune system; when working well, our immune system should clean up cancer cells and destroy them, before they ever get going as a tumor.

For this reason, you must be cautious with all "set diet" programs, even famous and supposedly successful ones, like the Gerson, Kelley or Burdwig programs.

Firstly, they may be working only by the exclusion effect (getting rid of likely problem foods).

Secondly, what they tell you are *good foods* may be toxic to you and produce a bad result.

In that sense, the *Diet Wise* plan is right for everybody, meaning each person should work out his or her own safe foods and stick to them. That is the lowest immune burden you can get and that's what you need, to maximise the fight against malignancy.

If you are battling this dangerous disease, be sure to read this book carefully and apply its important principles to your eating habits.

11

The Elimination Diet Step

This chapter and its procedure is the key to the whole success of the *diet wise* plan. Elimination dieting, that is the avoidance of certain foods as a means of recovery, was first pioneered as a technique by an American, Dr Albert Rowe Sr., as early as the 1920s. Many doctors have gone on since then to verify and extend his brilliant work. A classic text on this subject is *Food Allergy* by Herbert Rinkel, Théron Randolph and Michael Zeller, which dates from 1951.

Obviously, mere avoidance is not enough. A recovery might be coincidence. We follow through with a further step – introducing foods, one at a time, to test for adverse reactions. This is called "challenging." So the whole procedure we may christen *elimination and challenge dieting*.

I learned it from Dr. Richard Mackarness, the UK's great pioneer doctor, who had earlier written a successful diet book, *Eat Fat and Grow Slim,* which anticipated the Atkins low-carb diet by some fifteen years. Mackarness was a psychiatrist in a major British regional hospital and had put his patients through this regimen, sometimes with astonishing results. He wrote about these discoveries in *Not All in the Mind* (published in the USA as *Eating Dangerously).*

The elimination plan, given below, is simply a version of the Stone Age or "caveman" diet. Basically it consists of only meat, fish, fruit and vegetables plus water, with only slight modifications. Think of a caveman and his family walking through a forest or across the plains. They would eat fruit (berries etc.), gather roots (vegetables), occasionally catch fish or game; and they would drink only water.

It is important to remember that the exclusion diet is not for life, no matter how well you feel on it. Your maintenance diet may have a few exclusions but not all banned foods will turn out to be a problem. If not, you simply return them to your diet within a couple of weeks (after careful evaluation with a challenge test).

Fasting is the undercut

One logical way to find out whether you have food allergies or intolerance is to fast: if you stop eating and your condition clears up, there are few who would argue that food is incriminated. Surprisingly, most people feel terrific on a fast. Instead of being tired, miserable and hungry, the majority of patients report a zest and clarity of mind which they never knew or had forgotten existed. "I could have appeared on 'Mastermind,'" said one lady (meaning the TV program of the day; now superceded, I suppose, by "Who Wants to be a Millionaire?").

However you will be surprised to learn that I do not recommend fasting as an approach to the problem, no matter how logical. I have seen patients get into all kinds of difficulty with that method. Often, all foods will begin to react violently and getting back to any kind of safe eating platform is very difficult.

Some people should not fast on any account and to do so could be considered dangerous. The most obvious case is diabetes, where blood sugar control may be lost. But children should not fast, nor pregnant women or anyone in a very weak condition; neither should any person with schizophrenia or who has threatened or attempted suicide.

Only if you are robust and determined, preferably under the guidance of someone who knows the likely pitfalls of fasting, should you attempt this fast track approach. I will give you full instructions in Chapter 14.

Bowel transit time

The success of exclusion dieting rests on continuing for long enough to clear the bowel of all banned food residues. This usually takes about four days, but varies slightly from patient to patient. Thus it is possible to predict with a fair amount of certainty that symptoms will have cleared by the morning of the fifth day. Prior to that there are several days of 'withdrawal' symptoms, the severity of which again varies from one individual to another.

The masking phenomenon I have described depends upon a previous 'dose' of the foods still being in the body at the time of the next ingestion of that same food: thus at the end of the clearing period there are no more hidden allergies – not to food, at least. This is why the patient feels better.

The corollary to this is that there is no "masking" effect and any food now eaten will produce a marked reaction in accordance with the severity of the intolerance. We call this a *food challenge test* and the method I evolved over the years is the best I know. It often astonishes the unlucky patient to experience the full force of an adverse reaction to a food he or she had been eating almost daily, apparently without any ill effects.

The compromise

If you followed the explanation given above, you will have no difficulty in understanding how the plan works. In essence, it is a compromise with fasting: instead of avoiding all foods you are asked to omit only the *likely troublemakers*. The common allergy foods – a sort of 'top ten' – are wheat, corn, egg, milk, tea, coffee, cane sugar, yeast, citrus fruit (usually orange) and cheese. Others seem to vary according to consumption by the patient. For example, the tomato is quite a common allergen (although you would probably think it a fairly natural foodstuff), probably because it is consumed in such large quantities; we now eat winter salads, and tomatoes are very widely used in sauces and flavorings all year round.

Potato, from the same botanical family, may also have severe reactions. I have already remarked that for some reason it is a common cause of eczema – turning up far more commonly than it ought to. The fact is, as I have said repeatedly, any food can provoke symptoms. It varies from patient to patient. But short of banning all foods, which I have explained is not a good plan, the next best thing is to eliminate the most likely culprits. It's really about playing the odds.

I want you to follow this exact eating plan for ten to fourteen days. Maybe less: if your symptoms clear up entirely in the first five days, you can proceed to the next stage, which is the reintroduction of suspect foods, as described in chapter 12.

Foods you must avoid

To put this in reverse, the foods that you must avoid are as follows:

No grains: grains are the grass family (*Graminaceae*): wheat, corn, barley, rye, oats, rice and millet. Do not eat substitutes, such as spelt, which is really a kind of wheat.

This group of foods are very widespread in our diet. Wheat alone occurs in bread, cakes, cookies, muffins, pastry, pasta, as well as whiskey and many other distilled spirits. Corn is consumed as cornbread, hominy, grits, cereal flakes and sodas (corn syrup sweetener). Corn is a common binder in white tablets (pills), meaning a patient intolerant to it will react each time they pop a medication.

No dairy products; not even goat milk or sheep milk substitutes. The commonest allergy in this group is a protein called *casein*, which occurs in all milks. Dairy produce is also widespread in our typical diet and is often hidden from view. Milk, butter, margarine, cream, ice cream and yoghurt are obvious sources. But fruit juice may contain lacto-fermented whey, which is a dairy derivative.

No stimulant drinks. No tea, coffee or alcohol.

Quit smoking. You know you cannot seriously improve your health until you do.

Cigarettes are probably the most addictive of all the common social poisons. That is because tobacco is invariably a masked allergy. If you think back to when you first started smoking, the chances are that it made you quite unwell on the first few attempts (Stage I allergy), but you persisted and learned to tolerate it (Stage 2). Finally a condition of dependence was reached where too long a period without a dose produced withdrawal reactions (Stage 3): by then it started making you ill. But please understand this: I am not saying that unless you give up smoking this diet will not help you; it almost certainly will. Try very hard to stop, but if you cannot that is no reason to give up on your health – try the diet anyway.

Those afflicted with migraine and headaches should know of one very important statistic: half of all headache sufferers who stop smoking experience a dramatic improvement in their condition. Bear this in mind when you are next dying for a puff.

No sugar or substitutes, whether "natural" or synthetic. No white sugar, brown sugar or "natural sugar." Honey is not allowed, no *Stevia*, aspartame, saccharine or any other sweetener. *None of the allowed foods need sweetening.*

Give your taste buds a chance and get used to foods as they come. After a few days, even a carrot will taste very sweet.

Egg is not allowed. This is a wonderful strange food. Allergy to egg can be so exquisite that a patient kissing, or even shaking hands, with someone who has eaten an egg will react severely. It can happen that cutting a cake with egg in it and then using the same knife to cut an egg-free cake can lead to a skin eruption in someone super-sensitive to egg. *Ovalbumin* is the usual offending protein and occurs in all eggs. So turkey and duck eggs are not allowed in this initial phase.

Chicken is not permitted. This is not a matter of estrogens and antibiotics usually found in chicken (bad enough) but cross-reactions that can occur. Chicken and egg are, of course, the same animal effectively and sensitivity to one may mean a likely reaction to the other. You could eat capon (the male bird), if you live in a rural district and wish to take the trouble of tracking this down.

No citrus foods: that means no orange, lemon, grapefruit etc. At first this may seem strange. True there are many adulterated brands of orange juice, lemonade, etc. But the natural fruit should be OK, surely? Well, it's another of those empirical observations I made, meaning you just see it often enough to believe it. Orange (especially) can be trouble. As I point out to patients, the citrus family have very pungent odors: you can smell someone peeling an orange or lemon across the room. Powerful chemical substances such as this are the very stuff of allergy and intolerance reactions.

Last but not least: **no manufactured food of any kind**. Nothing from cans, jars, cans, bottles or packages. Nothing altered, "smoked" or flavored. Just eat your food as Nature made it.

It is hard for the layperson to grasp the criminal extent of adulteration of processed foods. Not only are essential nutrients removed, wholesale, but manufacturers will lie to you and try to pretend their product is "vitamin enhanced" or some such absurd claim. Consider this in terms of the story of a man walking down the street who is beaten up and robbed of $100. His mugger then returns $5 and says "Here you are; you're $5 enriched"!

But far worse are the atrocities put into food. Almost everything you can buy at the supermarket, other than organic fresh fruit and vegetable produce, has added chemicals. There are substances like polyphosphates, which absorb water and allow manufacturers to sell you water in pretence that it is a food ingredient. Bacon and ham may contain up to 45% water, which to my mind is simple legal fraud.

Other ingredients you will find if you care to investigate are anti-caking agents such as talcum powder (to stop food drying and looking like the crumbly nonsense that it truly is); emulsifiers which affect consistency; antioxidants, to retard the spoiling of fats; preservatives; and gelling or thickening agents.

Note all this is without even considering the thousands of chemicals that are used for flavoring and coloring. For years I kept a list of "apple flavor" chemicals to show patients; there are over eighty artificial substances, such as complex alcohols and esters, which go to make up the illusion of "apple." No real apple was included, of course. Just chemicals. To name just one: *(S)-2-methylbutanoic acid methyl ester* is a key ingredient for apple and strawberry flavor.

Cute words like "improvers" annoy me greatly. Such labels have nothing to do with the nutritional merits of the foodstuff. Take bread: an enhancer means a substance which will fluff up the bread to greater bulk, so that you buy more air for your dollars than would otherwise be the case. Note that bread may also contain chlorine and chlorine dioxide, metabisulfite and sulfur dioxide (the latter with water makes sulfurous acid, which is active enough to erode buildings of brick and stone).

BREAD

Often described as "the staff of life," bread is no longer the natural food it once was. The modern loaf or bun is so synthetic it remains plastic, soft and supposedly therefore "fresh" for days on end. I ask patients to consider the fact that mold will not grow on bread for many days, even when left exposed. If it is toxic to molds, I'm sure it is similarly so for humans.

Think of French bread – made fresh in the early morning but dry and inedible within a few hours. Wheat remains the number one toxic food, remember

---

"Natural" additives is another abuse of language. Food ingredients that may be claimed as natural are beetle cases, burnt feathers and seashells.

None of these additives are for the benefit of the consumer – they are added only in the manufacturers' interests. "But without them the consumer would not wish to eat the food," is the usual spurious argument in favor of additives. Well, hooray! would be my reply.

Beware the glutamate family

Processed food is really so denatured, bland and unpalatable that nobody would eat it, unless the flavor was "enhanced." The most common way of faking "flavor" is adding monosodium glutamate or one of its relatives.

Names to look for on the label are "hydrolyzed vegetable protein" and "modified vegetable starch." MSG and these similar compounds are all made by soaking rotten or otherwise unwanted vegetables in acid until they turn to brown sludge; caustic soda is than added to counter the acid. The final filth is added to what you eat from cans and packages, on the assurance they are "safe" and even "good for you."

Again there are lies galore: aware that most people nowadays are suspicious of MSG, manufacturers have taken to hiding its presence with labels that say "No MSG," "No MSG Added," or "No Added MSG," even though their products contain MSG and glutamate.

All this comes together in reinforcing my firm contention which is that you cannot trust food manufacturers. They will try to cheat and mislead you. *This is why I say on this diet plan, avoid all manufactured food. Don't take the risk.*

What to do about drugs, remedies and medications

Avoid drugs. By drugs I mean medicines, 'street' drugs, remedies, cures, tea, tobacco, coffee and vitamins. It is important to check with your doctor before abandoning any treatment he or she may be giving you, but do be alert to an authoritarian and unreasonable insistence that you do things his or her way: that way hasn't been working, or you probably wouldn't be reading this book. You therefore have a right to try any sensible alternative. The fact is that *very* few drugs are essential or life-saving. Insulin, thyroid hormones, epilepsy drugs, digoxin and one or two others spring to mind; the rest, such as painkillers, tranquillizers, antihistamines, antacids, sedatives, hormone replacements and the like are not strictly essential. Even the contraceptive pill, which is a steroid hormone, would be best omitted if possible.

The acid test is, how long have you been taking this drug? If you have been on it for years and are no better, it isn't really helping. At best it can be suppressing symptoms but not actually curing them. If you are taking any drug without really knowing why it has been prescribed, find out. Get your doctor to explain.

Don't be fobbed off with the usual 'You're too stupid to understand' attitude that a great many practitioners deplorably fall into (the ignorance is usually *theirs!*). If he or she is unable to sensibly defend prescribing the drug for you, don't take it. Many drugs are useless or cause complications, which seem not to worry the doctor but can make life unbearable for the patient. These side effects often result in the need for *another* drug to treat them, and matters can then become very complicated. I have on occasion seen individuals taking as many as eight or nine different drugs, several of which were to counteract the problems caused by the rest.

Often my patients have obtained immediate relief *simply by stopping all drugs*. I firmly believe that in a number of cases the original pathogenesis disappears and that the perpetuation of the illness is brought about by the continuance of the treatment, without anyone suspecting. This credibility gap is one of the reasons medical practitioners are fast losing face in the eyes of their own patients.

This is not meant as a criticism of my medical colleagues, though I admit it does sound like carping: the point is, you can just as easily be metabolically intolerant of drugs as you can of food and chemicals, so the very treatment you are receiving could be contributing to the problem. After all, there is no such thing as a harmless drug, no matter what assurances you are given. Thalidomide, which caused children to be born without limbs, was given extensive tests and hailed as safe, and was *especially recommended for pregnancy!* Vioxx, we all know, killed and injured tens of thousands of people before being withdrawn.

There will be others.

One of the problems with medicines is that it is not just the active compounds which cause trouble, especially for the allergy patient. Tartrazine, a commonly used yellow dye, is highly allergenic and yet responsible for the color of almost all yellow pills. Moreover, corn, a bad allergen, and other starches may be used for binding. There are numerous other ingredients, any one of which will cause a reaction, one example being HRT pills. One commonly prescribed product contains over thirty separate ingredients, only two of which are active hormones! Such 'cocktails' have almost inevitable consequences for the acutely sensitive allergy patient.

The last, and not the least important, reason you are asked to give up drugs is that you need to know what you are like off them and away from allergens. As I say to patients: if you are off your medication and no worse, that's real progress! If you are unable to give up your medication, go ahead with the diet anyway: improvement is perfectly possible and quite probable.

Incidentally, some of the above remarks explain why I also ban vitamins. Vitamin tablets are not dangerous in the same sense that drugs are, but these tablets also usually contain a great many additive ingredients that might be allergenic.

Casebook 8. Vitamin allergy

A thirty-eight-year-old woman went on a vitamin enhancement program which called for quite large doses. She rapidly became suicidal and had to stop. This was eventually traced to the niacin (B3) tablet, which was found to contain potato starch. Potato was known to have this effect, and she avoids it meticulously, but the tablets caught her out. This case, by the way, is one in the eye for those doctors who claim that patients 'imagine' their reactions to certain foods because they know they are eating them and so fake the symptoms. This woman had no idea, until she phoned the vitamin suppliers, that she had been eating potato.

You may not be taking *large* doses of vitamins, but this case is quoted to make the point: you may unknowingly be causing symptoms by taking *any* pills.

What about holistic remedies?

There is the question of homoeopathic remedies. It can be said with a fair amount of certainty that such remedies are not incompatible with this diet; however, the vehicle used can cause problems. The commonest of these is the simple white tablet. Known as Suc-Lac, it contains sucrose and lactose. You may recognize these as cane sugar and milk sugar, and you will readily see that these are *not* acceptable on the diet; neither is the plain white powder preparation soaked with the active ingredient, for that is also a sugar. Have a word with your homoeopath; tell him or her what you are doing. Most homoeopaths are very open to the subject of diet and nutrition. If you explain the problem, he or she should be able to provide you with a liquid to take as drops for this period.

It is important that you recognize herbal and other folk remedies as drugs; in fact, many plant extracts used as treatments were later found to contain quite potent drug substances, digitalis from foxglove being an example. When people tell me that herbs are natural and safe, I reply: "You mean opium, marijuana, hemlock?" This is not to compare the toxicity of modern drugs with that of simple folk remedies, but the fact is that no one knows the ingredients of most plant preparations. They *are* drugs and – more important from your point of view – they are certainly potential allergens.

In general, if you are in doubt, omit it. This is especially true if your 'cure' has been taken for any length of time. It obviously isn't curing you in any sense of the word, though it is possibly suppressing symptoms. You could probably manage it without it at least for the test period.

No stimulant drinks

Alcohol is banned on the exclusion diet. This is not being puritanical but because it too is a drug and has marked effects on the brain and body. Remember, if you are in any doubt, that rum was once used as an anesthetic for sailors when cutting off shattered legs. It is highly addictive, but worst of all it increases your allergy reaction to other foods also. Dr Théron Randolph, already mentioned, refers to alcoholic drinks as 'jet-propelled food allergies' – so be warned!

In any case, most alcoholic drinks contain substances that you will not be allowed to take on the diet (wheat, corn and sugar for example). What I usually say to patients is this: keep off alcohol until you are well. Then you can celebrate in champagne if you like – but be prepared to take the headache as a consequence! This is not a moral pronouncement against liquor but an entirely scientific one.

Next, tea and coffee. Make no mistake, these are powerful drugs with pharmacological effects on the heart, brain and kidneys. You must avoid them. Look around you at your friends or work colleagues: you will see an astonishingly high level of consumption of these drink substances. You should easily be able to spot the real addicts: they look anxious, restless and maybe even become short-tempered before the next "fix." As soon as they have indulged their craving they calm down again; you are observing a masked allergy.

Substitutes are not permitted, so decaffeinated coffee is *out*. Later, when you are well, you may be able to return to this drink: it is a big improvement on untreated coffee. But you will have to remember that the chemicals used to remove the caffeine will usually contaminate the final product and *may* cause you problems. Substitutes for tea are discussed

later, but all kinds of regular tea – China, Earl Grey, Formosa, Darjeeling and so on – are forbidden.

Permitted foods

Any meat: that means beef, pork, lamb; even rabbit, venison and other meats. Curiously, I found bacon and ham little problem in those years in the UK. However looking at typical American cured produce, with so many strange chemicals and flavors, I cannot recommend these products at this experimental stage.

Fowl. You may eat turkey, duck, quail and game birds (grouse and pheasant) if you are so inclined. You can even buy ostrich steaks on the Internet, from animals reared specially for the allergy market.

Any fish, and that means any fish or seafood in its natural state. Avoid smoked fish, even if properly smoked. Most of it, however, is not really smoked but treated with a synthetic flavoring. *Kipper brown*, for instance (also known as *brown FK* and *chocolate brown FK*) contains the following:

- 4-(2,4-diaminophenylazo) benzenesulfonate, sodium salt
- 4-(4,6-diamino-m-tolylazo) benzenesulfonate, sodium salt
- 4,4'-(4,6-diamino-1,3-phenylenebisazo)-di(benzenesulfonate), disodium salt
- 4,4'-(2,4-diamino-1,3-phenylenebisazo)-di(benzenesulfonate), disodium salt
- 4,4'-(2,4-diamino-5-methyl-1,3-phenylenebisazo)-di(benzenesulfonate), disodium salt
- 4,4',4-(2,4-diaminobenzene-1,3,5-trisazo)-tri(benzenesulfonate), trisodium salt

It's E-number is 154. (If a food additive has an E number this shows it has passed safety tests and been approved for use throughout the European Union.) It may also be used for salmon coloring and, as you may guess, for fake chocolate chips. It is currently banned in a number of countries, including Austria, Norway, Sweden, Finland, USA, Canada, Japan, Australia, France, Belgium, Spain, Portugal, Greece, Germany and Holland.

Any fruit except citrus. In modern supermarkets today there is a huge variety of fruits, some of them quite exotic and not available to us a few decades ago. Gone are the days when fresh fruit meant only apples, pineapple, bananas, oranges and grapes. Now we have kiwi, papaya, mango, Sharon (a variety of persimmon), star fruits, lychees, tangelos, exotic melons, Asian pears, and pluots to name just a few. Be adventurous. Think outside your normal habits.

All vegetables are allowed. This includes salad foods, naturally. Again, there is a huge variety of roots and leaves available in the modern supermarket. Colored ones are best (more antioxidants). But all have merits, even the flavor foods. Garlic is known for its antimicrobial and good cholesterol properties; chili has been shown to protect against bowel polyps (which are precancerous); cayenne pepper is good for arteries and the heart; curcumin (in turmeric) has advanced anti-cancer properties; so does onion; the list could go on and on.

Rutabaga (swede) mash makes a good substitute for the ordinary potato; butternut squash likewise. You can eat sweet potato (Spanish *batata*) or yams and these make nice fries if you cut them into penny circles and shallow fry. For a rice substitute, use cauliflower mash; you'd hardly know the difference, except visually.

Yes I know that 99% of vegetables are sprayed with chemicals many times before harvesting. But unless you are choosing the organic eating plan (more of that later), just tuck in and eat. Don't worry at this stage about the problems of storage, irradiation, nutritional content, GM variations or anything else. It's only for a couple of weeks.

Remember my key nutritional maxim: *what you are lacking isn't nearly such a big problem as what you are eating that you shouldn't.* This radical transformation of diet could be the most important health change you make in your entire life.

Certain canned or packaged foods are allowed. Very few, but these exceptions can be useful. Canned fish, such as sardines, salmon or tuna will be fine. Canned tomatoes too can be added to soups such as minestrone. Also frozen fish, vegetables and other foods. They may not be so nutritious or tasty but can be pressed into use when little else is available. Just make sure *nothing* is added and remember ingredients may not be listed: bisulfite is commonly used to sterilize vegetables or stop them browning, like pre-prepared fries, but would not be listed as an "ingredient."

Finally, for the purposes of this diet, dried fruit and nuts are OK, though a word of caution is needed. Most dried fruits are treated in some way. This usually takes the form of coating with mineral oil and bleaching with sulfur dioxide. These are substances to be avoided by choice, and it is better to buy at a health food shop run by knowledgeable people who can guarantee that their goods have not been subjected to this type of adulteration (I use the word 'knowledgeable' advisedly, because it is a sad fact that many health food shops are run by individuals who haven't a clue as to what they are selling!)

Salted peanuts and other packaged nuts are useless, as they contain additives. Get dry shelled nuts only. Again, the organically-oriented health food shop is the best place to find these. Otherwise buy a nutcracker and open your own.

Extras

A word on what we may call extras. Fried food is allowed. But do not use corn oil or any undefined oil, which may contain corn. Sunflower oil or safflower are good. Coconut oil is probably the healthiest, if you can master the taste. Olive oil is fine if you like Mediterranean food; remember not to heat it too high, otherwise it produces unhealthy smoke.

Salt and pepper are allowed but not sauces and condiments, like vinegar. For salad dressing, only oil and fruit juices are permitted.

Herbs are good and will help to keep the diet tasty. I have no problem with patients eating chilies and spices. They are all whole foods. Spices get a bad rap but I have invariably found that patients warned off them because of indigestion and other problems are fine. The real foods which inflame the stomach are wheat, dairy, coffee, sugar and so on. Once off these foods, patients can eat a full Tex-Mex or Indian curry and enjoy it without ill effects.

There are many surprises in store for you like this. Over the years I learned that most food wisdom handed around is faulty and better replaced by what you learn for yourself and about yourself!

Modifications

Now all that remains is for you to make any personal modifications. Look over your diet survey again. Try to be objective and decide if there are any foods that you eat rather a lot of which were not banned: these should also be excluded from the diet. It is hard to define what is meant by 'eating a lot of' a certain food; to some extent how you feel about it is a guide. If you are definitely keen on it and look forward to the next helping, take this as a warning of possible addiction!

For example, the common potato is often eaten excessively; many people don't feel the main meal of the day is complete without this vegetable. But do not underestimate its potential harm. I have seen a child lose virtually all its skin due to potato, a woman who spent twenty years in psychiatric care (including shock treatment) because of it, an Irish boy who almost went to jail for several years, because it made him violent, asthma cases and scores of other illnesses caused or made worse by apparently innocent helpings of mashed potatoes or fries.

Similarly, every daily food should be reviewed: just why are you eating it so repetitively? This is a question that should always arouse suspicion. *At least* reduce the frequency to one day in four as a safety precaution if you can't make up your mind whether or not to omit it altogether.

Will I be hungry?

No. This is not a slimming diet plan. You can eat all you want. It's just *what* you eat that is restricted, not quantity.

As I say to patients, if you are still hungry after a meal, cook it all again and eat it twice! Have ten meals a day if you want.

You get the point.

Even fried food is allowed. You can have French fries! That's good news.

By the way, you probably will lose weight. Most people do. Expect to shed about two lbs a week, without even depriving yourself.

Lots to eat!

Perhaps I should start by saying that you are not really restricted in reality – only in your own head.

There are a dozen readily available meats, if you are willing to eat rabbit and game.

There are several fowl other than the Fab Four (chicken, turkey, duck and goose): if you search the Internet there are at least three suppliers of ostrich meat to allergy patients, to which you can add quail, guinea fowl, squab, Cornish game hens, pigeon and doves.

The numbers of available fish reach the hundreds, though many are seasonal. Add shells and crustaceans and you have a huge variety of shrimps, prawns, crabs, langoustine, lobsters, clams, abalone and tasty nutritious foods galore. The added bonus is that omega-3 fatty acids from fish will help damp down the inflammatory response and so help any allergic or intolerant reaction.

Fruit was once very seasonal, as I remarked about Nature forcing rotation of our foods in Chapter 15. But today with supermarkets flying foods from all over the world to a counter just the next block from you, it is possible to buy plenty of fruits the whole year 'round. Moreover, supermarkets have sought to introduce their customers to exotic foods and there is no excuse for a limited parochial view. There are many hundreds of fruits to eat on a regular basis.

Then vegetables: much of what I just said about fruits is true for vegetables. Even northerly Maine is well able to raise a variety of edibles, including but not limited to: asparagus, beans, beets, broccoli, Brussels sprouts, cabbage, carrots, cauliflower, celery, Swiss chard, Chinese cabbage, pop corn, sweet corn, cucumbers, eggplant, endive, kohlrabi, kale, leeks, lettuce, muskmelons, onions, parsley, peas, peppers, pumpkins, radishes, rhubarb, rutabagas, spinach, squash, tomatoes, turnips and watermelons. I found several lists on the Internet and the consensus is that there are around 400 readily available vegetables for daily eating.

Out with the fluff

All in all there are well over a thousand readily available foods. So when patients say to me "What on earth is left to eat?" they get a sharp lecture in common sense.

Why would anybody miss eating the everyday foods, except because of laziness, habit and addiction? Bread, muffins, pastas, pastry and pizza are all wheat foods, with or without the yeast. Corn turns up in corn flour, most carbonated soft drinks (they use corn syrup as a sweetener), instant coffee, cornbread, polenta, pizza, pasta, tortillas, cornflakes and numerous other sugared breakfast cereals, cakes, cookies, muffins, waffles, instant desserts, ice cream, margarine, processed cheeses, jam, peanut butter, sandwich spreads, sausage, ham, bacon, wurst, variety meats, bolognas, popcorn, chocolate, chocolate 'flavor, chewing gum, sherbet, any dextrose-containing food, candy and chocolate bars, to name just a few. Even whisky, gin and most vodkas belong in this group – wheat (or corn) and yeast!

Corn, corn, corn. That's very *monotonous* eating in my book!

I am constantly astonished by the dismayed look I see when folks realize they are not allowed the usual breakfast cereals. You would think I was taking away their citizens rights! Yet to me these breakfasts-in-a-box are no better food or texture-wise than eating cardboard fragments.

When I suggest fish, liver, kidneys and chops instead, with fried vegetables, they look at me as if I said a dirty word. Yet to me this is a far healthier lifestyle breakfast. What's more the fat content blunts your appetite for many hours. There is absolutely no reason to be hungry on an exclusion diet. Try it and you'll see.

EXPENSIVE EATING

One thing is for sure, eating properly is expensive compared to eating junk. There is no denying this. Nor should it be a surprise to find that buying real food costs more than synthetic substitutes for the real thing.

It is a cost of living and cost of health that must be borne.

Remember though, this "test" phase of the diet is designed to last only seven to ten days; fourteen days at the outside.

What shall I drink on the elimination diet?

This is a natural and obvious question. Many people cannot imagine life without coffee, tea or a gin and tonic.

Water is the number one recommendation: spring water bottled in glass if you can get it (lots of scam waters; be careful). Perrier, Pellegrino and "designer waters" are fine, so long as they are pure.

Home filtered tap water may be even better, if you use the reverse osmosis. Do NOT use distilled water; it is denatured and lacks minerals (any rumored health properties are due only to the fact it is cleaner than normal water).

Certain fruit juices are permitted, also in moderation. These are apple, grape and pineapple, *not* orange and grapefruit. You must take care to get brands that say 'No additives.' Beware of cute manufacturers who say 'No artificial preservatives': they add what they claim to be 'natural' preservatives. This usually means lacto-fermented whey, and on a milk-free diet this is of course unacceptable. 'No added anything' is the kind of wording you should look for.

Herb teas are also allowed. These are plentiful and come in a great variety, such as matte, chamomile, peppermint or South African *rooibosch* (red bush). I do not recommend mixtures of flavors unless you are very careful. Many contain citrus zest and that would not accord with the elimination plan.

There are a few coffee substitutes on the market. While these may be useful long term, avoid these during the early test stage. Decaffeinated coffee is definitely not allowed. For one thing, it may have been chemically processed (methylene chloride or ethyl acetate). Also, under current federal regulations, a product can still contain 2.5% of the original amount of caffeine and be labeled "decaffeinated."

Seems tough?

I doubt if it is any worse than feeling ill most of the time. A lot of people find it surprisingly easy after the withdrawal phase is over. Remember, I am not suggesting that you eat like this for the rest of your life! It is a test designed to last ten to fourteen days. At the end of that time you should be able to draw definite conclusions. Often the results are quicker; maybe as little as five days. Sometimes, especially with 'slow' diseases like arthritis and eczema, you may need to be prepared to go on for longer.

The important thing is to bear clearly in mind that there are two stages of elimination dieting.

The first is this short stage, the *investigative diet*. It is demanding because you have to leave out a whole bunch of suspects at once. It is of little use to try and leave out foods one or two at a time. Think of Doris Rapp's eight-nails-in-the-shoe trap (page 43). If you pull out seven nails, you would still limp. You need to pull all eight nails, to get a result.

But once you have eliminated suspect foods and then re-introduced each one with a proper challenge test, as described in the next chapter, you will have only a short list of problem foods to avoid. You can stay off these long-term, by substituting other "safe" foods. This we can call the *maintenance diet*. You will find it relatively easy.

A lot of planning may be needed to bring about these changes in diet. As I say to patients, this will likely change your shopping habits, never mind your eating habits! It would be wise to locate suppliers of the items you need before getting started and stock the larder and refrigerator with entirely safe and allowed foods. I usually also recommend to patients that they *remove* from the house all the 'wrong' or banned foods: that way there is less temptation.

This may mean involving others in the household. I cover this topic of family co-operation later in the book.

You must be strict for it to work

For this exclusion diet to be a *valid* test you must perform it correctly. It is no good cheating 'just a little'. This is not a slimming plan where you can get away with an occasional indiscretion and still lose weight. Allergens work against you even in very small quantities: for example, think how minute traces of pollen in the atmosphere make hay fever sufferers so wretched in summer.

We are trying to clear *all traces of these particular* foods *from your body.* Only when you are totally free of a substance will you know if it has been upsetting you. When your bowel is clear of it, then it can no longer be a *masked* allergy; you will react on eating the food again, even if you never noticed it before. So you have two chances to catch the culprit: firstly, if you feel better for not eating it, that is a good clue; and secondly, if it makes you ill again after re-introducing it, that is as near to proof as you can get.

How we carry out these specific food tests is covered in the next chapter. In the meantime, just don't cheat – OK?

Breakfast - eat hearty

Breakfast seems to cause the most trouble. Take away corn flakes, tea and toast, and the average individual hasn't much of a clue how to start the day! Many people turn their noses up at the suggestion of fish, meat or fruit for breakfast. Some even look at me as if I had made an obscene remark. But look – if a food is healthy at six p.m. it is healthy at eight a.m. We don't usually eat haddock and fries for breakfast, but on this diet there is no reason why you should not (fish not battered, fries cooked only in sunflower or coconut oil).

Perhaps we have certain prejudices to which we would rather not admit. I once heard a man criticize a rather stuck-up middle-aged lady as belonging to the 'fur coat and kippers for breakfast set,' as if going without Corn Flakes or Rice Crispies were some dreadful upper-class affectation. I didn't tell him that for years I had been putting patients on fish breakfasts to solve the problem of low blood-sugar attacks! Herring is great; so are flounders, dabs or haddock! Fish roe tastes delicious, when in season, lightly fried with a little spicy pepper. Be a little adventurous: let your imagination run loose.

There is a very sound reason for eating a hearty breakfast, which I have just hinted at. If you eat carbohydrate, it tends to digest and dissipate quickly. This can lead to temporarily high blood sugar, which is over-corrected by the body, causing it to go too low. The victim recognizes this as tiredness and hunger and so is very soon eating again. Cereal and sweet things for breakfast (bread is a cereal food: wheat) set up this trap with a vengeance.

The best foods to protect you from hunger pangs are fat and protein; thus for your first meal of the day liver, kidneys, chops, fish and the like are a good investment against hunger and against the desire to stray from the diet and nibble 'snacks.'

The same enjoinder applies, though less forcefully, to your other daily meals. Eat heartily, and *don't* go *hungry*. Make a virtue out of breaking your normal routine. Others who continue to eat junk will be far more uncomfortable about your diet than you will!

Withdrawal symptoms

Let me now close this chapter with a reminder about withdrawal reactions. As with a junkie coming off heroin or an alcoholic who gets the DTs, the symptoms caused by stopping eating something to which you are addicted can be quite severe. Patients occasionally suffer so badly they have to give up working and retire to bed for a couple of days. It can be like this, but fortunately this extreme is rather rare: most people experience nothing more than a headache, tiredness and a disagreeable manner with friends and relations.

This unpleasant withdrawal phase has given rise to the fashionable and misleading term "de-tox" diet. Now that you are becoming *diet wise* you will better understand what is really happening on this step.

It *can* be a trying few days, and you must warn them it might happen or you will find yourself in conflict. It is especially important to be sympathetic with children in this phase; they are not being naughty as you might think, and to punish bad behavior would only add to the distress.

The point to remember is that if you do feel something out of the ordinary it is good news, so to speak: it means we have hit a bull's-eye somewhere. One or more of the foods you have ceased to eat was an allergen, and you are going to be correspondingly better in the long run. If that isn't comfort enough, then bear in mind that it will all clear up in a few days. Since, as I have said, it takes about four days to empty the bowel it is possible to predict that many cases, though not all, will wake up feeling refreshed and well on the morning of the fifth day. Patients are often startled by how accurate this is. Even if you vary by having symptoms that persist longer, your deliverance will come, so do persist.

The only exception to this last remark is the occasional individual who gets worse due to being allergic to something eaten on the diet – fruit for example. Again, this is rare and not a reason to give up when the going gets hard. Only if you are still feeling worse after ten or more days should you suspect you might be in this category. The way to deal with the problem is explained later (see Chapter 13).

Pronounced withdrawal reactions I usually treat by recommending a mild laxative such as Epsom salts or magnesia. The idea is that the sooner your bowel clears, the sooner you will feel better. If the reactions are very severe you probably won't feel like eating at all, and it is often a good idea to simply cancel all your engagements, relax with a good book and switch to a near fast of just grapes, yams, lamb and pears. This invariably cuts short the suffering.

Whatever happens, it is a good idea to remember that since food started it you will be able to sort it out using the information in this book.

Now that's enough of the preliminaries. Have a go and see what happens. *Bon appétit!*

12

What to Do if the Diet Succeeds

s I point out to patients, there can only be three outcomes for the exclusion test diet (after perhaps allowing extra time in certain situations): *you feel better, you feel worse or there is no change.* We will deal with each case in turn.

Best of all, of course, is feeling better. This is the usual case. If you met enough criteria from Chapter 10 which showed you were in an overload crisis and you properly simplified your diet as described, the chances are very high that you will feel really good. Maybe all symptoms have vanished.

Patient sometimes find a zest and energy they have not felt for years. Friends and family may even comment, "You look ten years younger!" It's one of my hearty sayings that the best treatment for a woman's complexion is diet! It far outweighs the artifice of creams and colorings.

All very nice.

But what if you have made only a partial recovery: Some of your symptoms are lessened, some have perhaps disappeared, and others remain unchanged? This is quite a common occurrence also and you should not be despondent: there are several more steps to go through after the preliminary diet which may bring further gains or possibly lead you all the way to a cure. What you have proved is that your illness has a basis in allergy or intolerance. For many people this will be the first sign of progress in years, and, of course, a degree of success. What follows is an attempt to build on this initial information.

You feel well

If you have recovered completely, then this is the easiest part of the book for you. Basically, what is required next is to identify those foods that were making you ill. We know there were several from the fact that you now feel better.

Incidentally, trouble foods rarely come singly. Many patients, I find, mistakenly expect to find one big troublemaker and that all the rest will be fine. This is not so: if you have developed one intolerance, you will almost certainly have several. Harris Hosen, one of the father-figures among American allergists, showed in a study of fifty consecutive patients that the average number of food allergies was between nine and ten per patient, though some had as many as twenty-five.

My own experience accords well with this.

How do we now pinpoint the correct foods? To do this you must eat each item under test conditions and see what happens. Those that cause symptoms are allergies and should be avoided. Any that appear harmless may be returned to your diet and continued with, as before.

We call this challenge testing.

Of course, like many patients, you may be feeling so much better that you don't want to hurry to change anything; you would rather not carry out any testing for the present. That is understandable.

But I'm afraid we cannot allow things to linger. The longer you stay off a food, the more likely the reaction will settle down. Even a gap as short as three weeks might be enough for the food to appear safe and pass the challenge test stage. That would be unfortunate because you would be led to believe it was a "safe" food, when in fact it would soon flare up and start causing trouble once more.

Think of a log fire that dies down to embers. It may glow very little and seem safe to put your hand in the ashes. But if you threw on more fuel you would soon see it burst into flame once again.

Patience is needed

Most of you, as I know from experience, probably can't wait to get off the diet no matter how much good it has done you. If you find it tedious and restricting, this is understandable. Yet a word of caution may be needed: the foods you miss the most and are so anxious to start eating again are very likely to be the ones that were making you ill in the first place. Don't forget that addiction and subsequent cravings are strong indicators of an allergy or maladaptation. You might be lucky in this respect; there are no hard and fast rules. But be warned: it will pay you to keep a tight rein on any residual longings you may have. You must dismiss from your mind the notion that you can simply go back to eating as you did before: something has to change, otherwise you will quickly become ill again. That 'something' is usually favorite foods eaten to excess. Such foods will in fact be reintroduced for testing *last of all.*

The correct thing to do is to start with what are probably harmless foods. Each new substance is tested carefully for safety, and those that cause symptoms must be rejected. Also, you must discontinue tests until the reaction has cleared up. This may be very inconvenient, so if you are in a hurry, that is all the more reason to proceed slowly. Milk and wheat (bread) are the most missed foods and, not by chance, they are in general the worst allergens. It is better to start with items such as chicken and rice first. These are rather less likely to provoke illness, and so there is more probability of expanding your diet without ill-effect.

Warning

The symptoms experienced when testing a food can be quite severe. It is unlikely that you will come to any actual harm but at times you may need courage and determination to go through with this procedure. It always comes as a surprise to patients when they realize what a bad effect a food causes, yet they had eaten it every day formerly without even suspecting it. This is because of the unblocking of the masking phenomenon. If you eat a food often enough, it will be permanently within your bowel. It is already in your body when you eat it again, so logically there is no reason for a response. Your body has learned to cope with the offending substance: it has *adapted.*

But when your bowel is completely emptied of that food you now have no protection and when you try to reintroduce it you will be hit with the full force of the negative reaction. Familiar symptoms will return with a vengeance. The correct thing to do, obviously, is to discontinue eating that food: the unpleasant reaction will disappear as soon as your bowel is once again cleared of it. This may take a few days. *During that time you cannot test any new food. You are stalled!*

You will see at once the wisdom of leaving the 'probables' (likely troublemakers) until last.

How to test a food

There is no infallible way of testing foods. The procedure given below is about as accurate as you can get and is a combination of methods pioneered by the American ecologists Herbert Rinkel and Arthur Coca plus my own recommendations. Follow it exactly and there will be very little chance of a trouble food slipping back into your diet by mistake.

If on testing you have a positive reaction, this is almost proof. Unusual false reactions may occur, but these can be sorted out later. Even then a reaction has *some* meaning; it might be that the method of storage or preparation induced some allergy capacity to the food that was otherwise innocent. If that is the case, then there is something useful for you to investigate anyway. Negative reactions are not so definite; nevertheless, you must make some assumptions, until proved wrong. Consider a food that doesn't react as safe. If you find yourself becoming confused, the best answer is to go back over the ground and test again.

My recommended procedure for individual food challenge tests

Test a food or drink only on a day when you feel well. It is no use testing food unless you are able to notice a reaction. If you are suffering from, say, a headache that day, how will you know if your test food causes headaches? True, it might make the one you've got worse. But that is too vague and risky. Having come this far, through care and diligence, why cut corners? Wait for a better day.

1. Test only at lunchtime. I realize that this can be difficult with children who go to school, but there is a good reason for choosing this meal instead of others. It isn't always easy to tell first thing in the morning whether the day is a good or a bad one for you, but by lunchtime you should know for sure either way. Avoid testing at breakfast unless you feel bright and sparkling (some people *are* like that at the start of the day, believe it or not!).

2. Testing at your evening meal is not wise: most symptoms come on in the first few hours, and you might have a reaction in the night when you are asleep and miss it. This could spare you a little discomfort, but you may be misled as to the results of the test and become confused.

3. Eat only the food you are testing at the first test meal. Take a reasonable portion, for example two apples, half a pint of milk or two slices of bread (no butter). Sea salt may he used if needed; not

table salt. Spring water is allowed – nothing else. It is important, if you have a reaction, to be quite sure that the test food caused it. You cannot have this degree of assurance if several items were eaten at one sitting. If you eat just the one food and within a few hours feel ill, then the cause was most likely that food, or not a food at all.

4.   Eat the food raw or prepared very simply. Cooking can alter the reactivity of food. For example I found over the years that well-cooked beef usually has more adverse effect than the same joint or cut when underdone. Minced, chopped or ground food is also more likely to react: breaking it up speeds digestion and in effect increases the absorption. Frying on the other hand tends to slow down a reaction, probably because the fat coating holds back the body's contact with the reactive substances.

5.   If you have no observable reaction during the afternoon, include more of the test food with your evening meal. No symptoms that day or by next morning mean that the food can generally be regarded as safe. *Most reactions, luckily, take place fairly quickly, often within an hour. Note that the symptom may begin fairly mildly soon after testing and only reach full force hours or even days later. It is when it first comes to your attention that counts: whatever you ate just before that time is the culprit.*

6.   Take a pulse count. You can increase the accuracy of this procedure considerably by including a simple pulse count. Arthur Coca showed in the 1950s that allergic exposures may alter the pulse rate; it was actually his wife who had first commented that her heart raced after eating certain foods. Historically, many interesting discoveries have come out of chance observations of that sort. Credit is due to Coca, of course, for having the acumen and curiosity to pursue the finding.

The correct way to include this extra information is to take your *resting* pulse shortly before eating a test food. By 'resting' I mean sit down for at least two minutes. If you have been engaged in any strenuous exertion, allow five minutes. Count for a full sixty seconds; don't do as busy nurses do and count for fifteen seconds then multiply by four, as for our purposes that isn't accurate enough.

After eating the food, take a repeat pulse count at intervals of twenty, forty and sixty minutes. Keep a note of the results. (It isn't necessary for you to sit still for the whole hour, merely for a couple of minutes before the reading.) A rise *or fall* of ten or more beats per minute at any of these intervals is very strong evidence that you are allergic to the food being tested, even if you get no symptoms. If the pulse does not rise, that doesn't mean you have no allergy. And, of course, if you do experience symptoms, *even if the pulse rate does not change,* that means you are allergic to the test item.

7. Test with organic foods if you can get them. By organic foods I mean those grown in a natural way, without chemical additives or contaminants, such as crop sprays, and sold without packing or preservatives. Apples from a neighbor's garden, if the season is right, are better than the commercial variety. A chicken that has been reared free range, without chemical additives to its feed, such as antibiotic (which is used to keep battery birds 'healthy' in unsanitary, overcrowded conditions) is better than the supermarket equivalent. Unrefined food should be used instead of pre-cooked or packaged versions.

    If you can't get the ideal food, go ahead and carry out your tests anyway; use whatever you can obtain without unreasonable demand on your resources. But it is vitally important that you be alert to the implications of the contamination of commercial food sources, otherwise you will draw the wrong conclusions. For example, you may think you had a bad allergy to cabbage when in reality it was the heavy chemical residue on the leaves caused by the crop's being treated with fungicide and insecticide that made you ill. This is still perfectly valid information: it means that if you can't get cabbage free of this pollution, you must avoid it. But it might be nice to know that you *could* eat cabbage now and again, providing it comes from a safe supply! (See appendix B.) Cabbage has just been added to the Environmental Working Group's list of "clean" foods.)

8. Reject all dubious foods, at least for the moment If you think you reacted to a food, it is no use saying to yourself, 'I'll try again tomorrow'; by eating the food as a test you have probably masked any reaction for several days. In this interval you may eat the food and learn nothing because this does not mean it is safe for you. Better to delay for at least five clear days – longer if you are constipated.

In the meantime, get on with testing other foods. The second time around you may get a more definite answer, yes or no. If it remains doubtful avoid it altogether, at least for ten to twelve weeks; then try again.

As a final point, you can try testing foods prepared in different ways. Cooking, for instance, both creates and destroys allergens. If you can't take a food raw, try cooking it and repeat the test (at least five days later).

ANIMAL BEHAVIOR

It is interesting to observe that animals will usually test their food carefully, before eating it. Notice how a dog sniffs and then licks its food, to check it. Only if satisfied that the food is safe and wholesome will the dog go ahead and eat all the food.

How unlike humans; we know that certain foods are bad for us – some foods even smell or taste synthetic and unpleasant – but we go ahead and foolishly eat them anyway.

There is psychology in this too. Before you eat, you should picture how you will feel thirty minutes after consuming the food. Often you know very well you will feel bloated, stressed and wish you hadn't.

Well, don't do it! Change your approach…

What to do if you experience a reaction

As I said earlier, if you don't react to a food it is moderately sound evidence of adaptation. If you *do* react, on the other hand, it is pretty definite that you are maladapted (intolerant) to that food. Neither outcome is proof positive, but providing you follow the above procedure closely you should be able to rely on the results. A reaction may mean either a single symptom or that you feel quite ill with many. Regardless of how mild or severe it is, you must wait until this clears up and you feel well again before proceeding with further tests. This may be irksome, but is necessary in accordance with the first point of the procedure outlined above.

Recovery can usually be speeded up by taking a mild laxative.

Epsom salts, one or two teaspoons in half a glass of warm water, are recommended. Do not take syrups or compounds at this juncture; you have no idea what ingredients they contain. In addition, it has been demonstrated that an alkaline salts mixture helps. It is probable that the body fluids swing towards acidity during an adverse reaction, and this helps to correct the balance.

> You can easily make up the formula for yourself. Mix one part potassium bicarbonate to two parts of sodium bicarbonate. Take a dessertspoonful of the resulting mixture in half a glass of water. Few pharmacists nowadays stock potassium bicarbonate – most of them are given over to prepared drugs and cosmetics – but if you persist you will find one. Incidentally, don't overdo this last remedy, even though it seems to work like magic: excess alkalinity is as bad as acidity and has its own dangers and problems.

I'm sure you will recognize in the above two tried and true old-fashioned 'cures,' yet they do work well. I'm convinced that many cases of passing gripes and collywobbles in years gone by were due to incompatible food reactions, though no one would have recognized them as such. But our ancestors did hit on the right remedy without realizing how or why it worked.

Delayed reactions to foods

Most allergy reactions to foods come on within one to twelve hours, in other words quite rapidly. Some are even quicker and, not infrequently, patients report an *almost instantaneous* effect when eating a food. Up to twenty-four hours is not uncommon, where for example, something eaten one morning appears to be responsible for a symptom that is present on waking the next day.

Much more rarely, however, it appears that a food can cause *delayed reaction:* that is, the symptoms do not appear for over twenty-four hours, even for up to forty-eight in exceptional cases. This is especially true if the individual continues to eat that food, and I have often heard patients describe this situation as a 'build-up.' It is important to be aware of this effect when you are carrying out tests, or you may come confused.

Suppose you were testing milk and there was no observable reaction. 'Good,' you might think, 'I'll carry on taking milk in my diet.' This is quite proper. The next day you might test egg, and again there is no response: at the same time you are having milk. On the third day you might introduce pork and feel ill: obviously, it was the pork! Well, *it may not have been if you are having a delayed reaction to milk*. If this does happen to you, it can become very confusing. You may be ill again before you know where you are and have learned nothing about your allergies. What do you do? Well, the thing *not* to do is give up.

Think of the delayed reactions if you do not get well rapidly after avoiding a test food that caused a return of symptoms, especially if you used the bicarbonate remedy given in the previous section. The reason could be that you are not avoiding the right food. Go back to three days *prior* to the re-onset of symptoms and eliminate all foods introduced since then. Recovery within two to four days will confirm that delayed reactions are the problem.

If necessary, go back to the elimination diet exactly as given. You were well (or much better) on it, so always revert to it in a crisis or when you find yourself stuck for an understanding of what has been happening. This becomes your default position or baseline for wellness.

If you do stumble and find yourself floundering with uncertainty, proceed with tests much more slowly: instead of trying a new food each day, introduce only one or at the most two items a week. Eat them regularly each day in substantial quantities and see if you can force a reaction.

If after four days of eating something fairly intensively you feel no different, then it is indeed a safe food. You may then proceed to the next one. Don't continue to eat the safe food in abundance, by the way, otherwise you may develop a reaction to it even if you don't have one at the time of testing: moderation is the key to food indulgence and staying healthy (see Chapter 15).

What to do if no food reacts on testing

Even more rarely, it may happen that nothing seems to react when you perform challenge tests. This is puzzling because, having felt better avoiding certain foods, you would naturally assume that one or more of them wasn't suiting you. This is a logical deduction and one that remains quite valid.

The reason for this anomaly is that avoidance of an allergen, even for as short a period as two weeks, can reduce the fierceness of the sensitivity to a point where a single test dose, or even a series of meals containing the food, becomes insufficient to provoke the response from the body. The reaction has died down.

In order to understand this better it is necessary to know something about fixed and cyclical allergies.

Fixed allergies. As the name suggests, these are unchanging. No matter how long the food is avoided, the response will remain the same. The late great Theron Randolph of Chicago considers that an allergy should not be designated 'fixed' unless, after two years' *strict* abstinence from it, the food still shows a propensity to create symptoms.

Fixed allergies tend to be severe and are the type, such as peanut sensitivity, that might easily give rise to an anaphylactic reaction. It is a lifelong affliction, but fortunately this is the comparatively rare type.

Cyclical allergies. These are more usual. Basically, sensitivity to food is a function of the frequency with which it is eaten. The more you come into contact with the substance, the worse the reaction gets; the less contact you have with it, meaning in terms of *frequency* rather than quantity, the more the sensitivity will subside. Complete avoidance of the substance may mean that ultimately there is no reaction to it at all. Nevertheless, the *potential* remains: in the case of an offending food, if it is again eaten often, the allergy will flare up.

This phenomenon of cycles was first noticed by Herbert Rinkel, who used it to devise rotation diets whereby the patient ate a given food only at set intervals infrequent enough to prevent the build-up of a cyclical allergy. It is possible that through avoidance of an allergen, the reaction will settle down in as few as ten to fourteen days. Thus testing it after such an interval may give the impression it is a harmless food, whereas in fact it was one of the causes of the initial illness. Nevertheless it must be emphasized that re-adaptation is rarely so rapid: several months are normally required.

Two plus two is more than four!

The second reason you may not find obvious reactions to foods is because of the summation effect.

It happens sometimes that none of the substances consumed cause much effect on their own. If they react at all it is so mild the patient never notices or does not care. You may, for instance, find eating ice cream give you mild bellyache sometimes – not enough to stop you enjoying the occasional scoop.

Trouble comes, however, when foods fall in certain combinations. Some have a tendency to interact with each other and cause definite symptoms when in the right (wrong) combination.

As with drugs when administered together, it is possible that the combined effect of two is more than twice the effect of each singly, perhaps many times more. This is called *potentiation*. You may have heard that a combination of alcohol and barbiturates can be fatal even in modest doses. This is a poor example because it comes from the world of garish murder stories and television 'thrillers,' but it happens to be quite valid. It is an instance of potentiation, and food intolerances may behave in the same way.

I sometimes use the example of an hypothetical individual allergic to cats, dust, chocolate and milk. All may be well until one day he drinks a chocolate milk shake and then strokes a cat in a dusty attic: at that moment all four allergies come into play, and he sneezes. The victim carelessly observes: "I must be allergic to cats."

But without the milk there may have been no sneezing. If he tested himself with the chocolate, milk or dust, nothing would appear untoward. In general he has no symptoms, but next time he strokes the cat nothing happens and this might be puzzling. Another day he has a glass of milk and a bar of chocolate quite close together and develops a runny nose. But there is no cat in sight, and now he doesn't know what is wrong; he hasn't heard of food allergies anyway, and thinks he's getting a cold! It is only when all the allergens occur together that sneezing occurs.

So it can be with food. You may observe no particular reaction on performing individual challenge tests, yet slowly you deteriorate and revert to your original condition. This is because moderate food intolerances are potentiating one another.

If you suspect this situation, then go back to the elimination diet until you feel well. Then proceed as for delayed reaction testing, allowing several days between each new food. As soon as you begin to feel less than optimum, suspect the last combination. Say you introduced bread the first week, egg last week and milk this week and that you are now noticing something is wrong. Suspect the egg/milk combination. Instead of stopping the milk, stop the egg. If it clears up, it means that egg and milk together don't agree. Obviously, milk is tolerated – you got well again while still drinking it. Egg alone was also OK because you ate it for a whole week with no ill effect. (In this example, if you *didn't* recover by stopping egg I'm sure you can deduce that either milk *must* have been the culprit or the culprit is not a food at all.)

By applying the above principles you may be able to work out several combinations of foods that don't suit you; simply avoid them. Nevertheless you should study Chapter 15 with particular reference to the section on rotation diets, as you will almost certainly need one of these.

Keep a food diary

Throughout this plan it is a good idea to keep careful records. One type of record that will be very helpful we call the food diary. At times this will help you to work out what has been happening to you, and it may also reveal useful pointers to allergens if you know what to look for. Take an ordinary notebook and divide the pages in half with a vertical line. Date each page, and in the left-hand column write down everything you ate and also any important activities. Foods should be listed by meal and the time of the meal entered also; include details of how it was cooked.

On the right-hand side of the line write down any changes in your condition. If a symptom starts up, jot it down with the time. It may also be important to note when a symptom disappears. Now you will see the value of keeping a note of times.

If, say, a headache appears at about 2:00 p.m. you would notice that lunch was at 1:15 p.m., and the foods included in that meal immediately became suspect. On the other hand, if the headache *started* at 1:05 p.m. you would ignore lunch and concentrate more closely on breakfast.

The diary will do a great deal to help pinpoint likely troublemakers. For instance, if you were fairly certain which meal was to blame, the most likely food in that meal would be one which you had not eaten for at least four days; this would mean it was unmasked at the time of eating. Count backwards and check which ones qualify – get the idea?

Cultivate the diary. Keep it with you wherever you travel and make sure it is up to date: it can be very disconcerting to have a reaction and find you cannot remember what you ate because it wasn't written down at the time. This isn't meant to make you paranoid about your diet, by the way – just keep everything in perspective. The food diary is a temporary tool; a short-term means of regaining full health. Don't be obsessive.

How long do I avoid allergy foods?

Once cyclical allergies have been explained, most patients realize that it is not necessary to stay off allergy foods permanently. After a due interval some of these foods will be found adapted to once again and be easily tolerated in the diet provided they are taken in moderation. As with so many things, it depends on the individual case.

If you make a rapid and thorough recovery you may be in such good shape that you are able to try out the implicated foods within two to three months. But for most people this would be far too soon; six months is a safer interval; maybe a year.

In any case, no food should be returned to your diet without being subjected to the rigorous procedure of challenge testing outlined earlier in this chapter. Even then, if you seem inexplicably worse off, remove the latest food addition at once; do not continue eating a food that causes you to feel even slightly less than optimum – because it will only get worse. Remember, merely eating the food tends to generate reactions.

Be patient and you will be rewarded. Allergies don't disappear overnight, and it will almost certainly take a long time. But if you tackle the problem sensibly you *may* be able to return to eating some of your favorite foods. Just never lose sight of the fact that these once made you ill and can do so again.

Staying well

Once you have traveled this far you should be very pleased. By now I expect you will be feeling much better, if not completely well, and have a catalogue of foods that disagree with you.

If success is not yet complete, or there is no result, the next chapter may contain information that may pave the way to it. Also, remember there are causes for disorder other than food allergies, such as environmental allergens, hypoglycemia, hyperventilation, parasites and Candida (which we shall learn more about in chapter 21).

If you feel fine, now would be a good time to consider vitamin and mineral supplements to build up your defenses. As I said earlier in the book, allergies and intolerance may well be due to deficiencies of these vital substances since they act as enzyme precursors.

SUMMARY

If you felt partially or wholly better on the elimination diet, there were important allergens amongst the foods you gave up.

- Alternatively, you may want to wait for a few months and then try the foods again

- From then on follow the procedure for testing and any food that passes may be allowed cautiously back into your diet. passes.

- Never over-indulge in a food that has once caused a reaction.

- If you start to feel worse, you have recommenced eating an allergy food that you shouldn't have. Simplify your diet until you feel well and proceed cautiously with the reintroduction of foods.

- Staying well is not the same as getting well, and you are referred to Chapter 15.

- Vitamins and minerals help in the fight against allergies. Even whole foods may be deficient in these substances, so consider supplements.

13

What to Do if the Diet Fails

I f you feel no different on the diet, or perhaps even feel worse, do not at this stage assume you have no food allergies; in fact, if you feel *worse,* that might be good evidence that you do. The probability is that you are eating much more of an allowed food which disagrees with you. No food is absolutely safe. If, for example, you are allergic to certain meats or fruit, then you are hardly likely to feel well on my exclusion diet!

Fortunately, few people feel worse on the diet; but if it happens this can yield useful information. How to proceed in that event is described below. If you are already aware of an item that you are consuming heavily, suspect that item and proceed immediately to the modified test procedure a few pages hence. If nothing seems obvious, keeping a food diary for a few days (as directed at the end of the previous chapter) should yield plenty of suspicious candidates for testing.

As stated earlier, one prime culprit I find from my practice is potato. It is a staple that is consumed heavily, daily in most British people's diets, and so, not surprisingly, quite a common allergy. When patients are prevented from eating their 'normal' quota of bread, cakes and carbohydrate 'fillers' as they tend to be christened, potato becomes the only available substitute, and it is not unusual to find people eating it twice, even three times a day while on the elimination program.

Casebook 9.

It is far from being harmless: I have seen several very severe cases of potato intolerance. I have already reported the case of a little boy of eighteen months with life-threatening aczema due to potato (Casebook 6, page 90). Years later an unfortunate lady I recall came to see me with severe eczema;in in fact it was so bad she had a virtual "open ticket" at the local hospital, allowing her to check herself in when things got too bad. On occasion she would report with her clothes stuck to her skin, oozing blood, and sheets of dead skin would come away as her clothes were soaked and peeled off.

Very dramatic, I dare say. But actually an easy one. Potato was just about the only significant food reaction I found and if she stayed off it, she was fine!

Another case concerns a woman who had severe psychiatric problems. For over twenty years she had been ill and had numerous major antidepressant drugs and courses of shock treatment in an effort to treat her condition, all to no avail. She turned out to have a potato allergy. It was her habit to consume, with her husband, some 3 lbs. of potatoes daily! Remember what was said about food addiciton in chapter 7.

Once off potato and the rest of the nightshade family the woman was fine (potato belongs to a fairly toxic food family called the nightshades (after Deadly Nightshade *Atropa belladonna*). Chili, peppers, tomatoes and eggplant are in the same family; so is tobacco!

You felt no different

When correctly chosen for the elimination diet, about seven out of ten cases improve, one feels worse and the other two feel no change whatsoever. The first point to check, if you are in the latter category, is, do you qualify? The self-inventory in Chapter 10 is designed to establish this. Perhaps you should look over the points again. The more positive answers you give to the table of symptoms, the more certain it is that we are dealing with an allergy or intolerance. It may not be food: chemicals sensitivity and inhaled allergens can have an equally devastating effect.

Stress too can prevent recovery from health problems. If your life is off balance and not giving you what you want: that's stress. There is abundant evidence that stress underlies almost all negative health conditions. Maybe you need to make significant changes which bring you closer to what you want. At the very least move out of the need zone. If you can't immediately get all you desire for a happy life, you can surely relax and stop giving yourself a hard time about what you're missing. Consider a change of job, a change of relationship or even just a change of attitude, to bring you closer to contentment.

In the meantime, finish the review given below...

Did you carry out the diet correctly?

This is a vital point: if you didn't do it exactly as written you may have denied yourself the beneficial result. This is not like a slimming plan in which you can cheat just a teeny bit and it doesn't matter. You must remember what we are trying to do, and that is to clear your bowel *completely* of the suspect foods. If after four days of being careful you then slip up and eat something forbidden, it means that we have to wait another four or five days for it to clear. In the meantime you may make no recovery, and we shall learn nothing. If you lapse again in this manner, you'll get nowhere.

So – did you stick to it *rigidly?* This isn't a moral or character-building point but a very practical one.

One of my patients is so sensitive to tomatoes that he cannot enter a room where they are being cut up without having an immediate asthma attack (incidentally, he was eating them regularly when we commenced the plan but the severity of the condition was completely masked). I have several cases of individuals who cannot touch an egg, or even handle an object that has contained egg, without getting a skin eruption. These are, needless to say, extreme cases. I am only making the point that *quantity is unimportant*, tiny amounts count, therefore lapses may defeat the whole plan.

It does happen that certain individuals feel better even if they restrict foods carelessly and make mistakes. But they are lucky; you mustn't count on chance. It is more scientific to *make* things work in your favor. Nothing could be more disappointing than to struggle through two weeks of deprivation only to find you did not get well because of carelessness.

You might even be misled into thinking that you were not a food allergy or intolerance case and miss the very cure that you are seeking. If you have not followed the diet correctly you have little choice other than to start again and follow it as written for *at least seven more days* before making up your mind as to the result. If you *then* feel no better, you may assume that the diet did not help and proceed as given in this chapter.

Bowel transit time

Sometimes what prevents success is that the bowel is sluggish. Food may take as long as two to three weeks to pass through, even when stools are evacuated each day. Ironically, the bowel can be stuffed with old hardened food residues, while food eaten later hurries past. Of course, foods will not unmask properly if they are present in the bowel. This can make matters very confusing.

If you suspect this difficulty, you may be able to detect it by a *charcoal tablet test*. Swallow six or eight charcoal tablets, which are obtainable from the pharmacist. Then time how long it takes before the charcoal first appears in your stools and also when it last disappears.

The record at my office so far is three weeks (slowest) and ninety minutes (fastest).

Individuals with below average transit time should add another week or more to the trial period, before deciding that the test diet has not been effective.

Testing the banned foods

Just because you feel no better on the elimination step does not mean that you cannot be intolerant to any of the banned foods. This is an important point.

Recovery may be denied you because of foods you are still eating. The list of allowed foods is really only playing the odds: they are the most likely offenders. That's all. It is perfectly possible to be allergic to meat, fish, fruit or any of the allowed foods. They are permitted because this is not so common, that is all.

If you remove one or two foods that you react to but continue to eat others which are a problem, there may be no apparent change in how you feel. So never assume that the banned foods *must* be safe, just because you do not feel better avoiding them.

But how can we test these foods by challenge testing, if you have not eliminated your symptoms? There is a problem. You can tackle it one of two ways, depending on your temperament and determination.

The tougher alternative would be to give up even more foods, to see if you can get to a point of fewer or no symptoms. Then proceed as before. An easier alternative is to go ahead anyway, challenging the banned foods, in the hope that symptoms will show up among those already present. Existing symptoms may worsen or fresh symptoms will appear at the time of testing. After many years, I can tell you that it does sometimes work this way.

A positive reaction is, after all, still positive. It is only when you are vague or feel no different that a food which shouldn't can slip through the net. The thing to do is to mark your notebook to that effect so that you can always come back to the food in question and test it again, supposing that we arrive at a stage where symptoms are either reduced or have disappeared completely.

Modified test procedure

If you are determined and want to reduce the diet further, it would be logical to try to detect the foods that are continuing to cause you problems. Some of this is guesswork; some, as you will now know, is based on frequency of consumption. Foods you eat only rarely are not what we are looking for.

There will no doubt be a number of allowed foods that you eat daily, as you have always done. What about potato? Onion? Tomato? Lettuce? Don't suppose salad foods are healthy for everyone. Lettuce is a surprisingly common offender, resulting in illnesses from migraine to colitis. Don't get caught out.

Set yourself a program of testing each one in turn. It is logical to start with those you consume most of or, more exactly, consume most often: overindulged foods are always prime suspects.

Avoid the food for five days and then challenge it.

Of course if you feel better soon after dropping it out, that's a good sign and you will be particularly careful to nail it when carrying out the challenge test.

Omitting groups of foods

It is possible to exclude different groups of foods to those banned on the Stone Age diet. If up to this point you have not succeeded, you might like to try omitting each of these groups in turn. A number of suggestions are given below.

Meat-free

Not everyone feels much better as a vegetarian, but you have only to read the success stories of some people who have adopted this lifestyle to realize that it suits quite a number. We can deduce that these people must have been allergic to meat in some form or other. Unfortunately, many more people are allergic to grains and dairy produce than to meat. This is sometimes hard to get across to vegetarians, who tend to be enthusiastic campaigners. It means, in effect, that fewer people are suited to vegetarianism than are made ill by it. This is an overall view, which does not take into account individual cases. Where vegetarianism *does* help is that it tends to be part and parcel of a movement towards whole foods and away from manufactured and 'junk' food. Inevitably this is associated with increased health and vitality.

Casebook 10.

To illustrate the point I am making, let me describe the case of a young woman in her late twenties who came to see me because of asthma. At college she had become interested in health foods, healing and the occult; she then decided to be a vegetarian. For a long time this apparently suited her and harmonized well with the way of life she and her friends led. However, while engaged in full-time study, she began to notice that her mental faculties were not as good as she knew them to be.

Things got worse. She became drowsy and apathetic; her brain wouldn't clear in the morning and she tended to forget what she was doing, even where she was at times. As the listlessness grew worse, she became unable to attend college and at one stage ended up in a zombie-like trance that lasted many weeks. She would lie in bed, out of touch with reality and, to the despair of her friends, rising only occasionally to eat a little food, perform her natural functions and go back to bed. This continued day after day for almost three months.

Then she had what she described as a vision of a fish and realized that Nature was telling her she should eat some. This she did, and felt a little better. That prompted her to try eating meat, and from then on she improved rapidly: Within a matter of weeks she was her old self, resumed her studies and graduated successfully in the normal time.

It is remarkable – and perhaps fortuitous – that students living away from home can experience such ill health and that it can remain undetected. As it was, she had a lucky escape. It is no exaggeration to say that, like so many allergy patients, she might have ended up as a lifelong, institutional case in a psychiatric ward without anyone suspecting the real reason. Instead, a lucky change of diet cured her.

All this emerged in the course of our discussions about her asthma, which she suffered from quite badly. Testing under my care showed that she was severely allergic to the grains. Even today, if she exceeds one slice of bread in twenty-four hours her mental condition deteriorates markedly, and a real binge drives her out of touch with her surroundings to an alarming degree. Yet for years she ate heavily of the grain family, as vegetarians often do. Undoubtedly this built up her cyclical allergy to wheat, and her excursion into meatless eating was almost a disaster.

Nevertheless, some people are made ill by beef, pork or lamb (rarely all three in fact). Commercial meats often have chemical contaminants of some kind, such as hormones and antibiotics. It is a practice with some suppliers to treat meat with agents to keep it red; niacin, also known as vitamin B3, is such a substance. That could be healthy, you might suppose, and so it could; but niacin is notorious for the side effect it produces of a burning flush, rather like being exposed too long in the sun. If a hearty steak tends to do this to you, perhaps it is really the 'harmless' vitamin pollution at work!

Include a two-week meat-free regime in your self-assessment program. If there is any improvement, find out which meats by reintroducing them as before.

Pulse-Free

The elimination diet, or Stone Age diet, is in effect grains-free, dairy-free and chemical-free with a few refinements, such as no sugar and stimulants. Next to these foods, the pulse family is arguably the commonest group of troublemakers. These are also called legumes (peas and beans). It should not be forgotten that peanuts (a bean, not a true nut), lentils and soya (often used as textured vegetable protein, TVP) are also members of this botanical group.

There are a great many biological toxins to be found in pulses, which means that most of them are poisonous unless cooked particularly well. This could account for the fact that, as a family, they are not always well tolerated.

After your meat-free experiment, try two weeks pulse-free.

Nut and pip-free

Some people don't tolerate fruit very well; with others, nuts are a problem. This may be a sign of allergy to the birch tree pollen (*Betula* species). Foods to avoid in this group are almond, apple, apricot, raw carrot, raw celery, cherry, coriander, fennel, hazelnut, kiwi, nectarine, parsley, parsnip, peach, pear, peppers, plum, raw potato, prune, tomato and walnut.

These may be foods to suspect if you felt *worse* on the Stone Age Diet. You probably increased your intake of these foods. Try eliminating them now as part of the program.

A larger group exclusion we call the "nut-and-pip-free diet": tomatoes, apples, plums, nuts, marzipan, coconut, pears, plums, cherries, bananas, pineapple, peas, apricots, peaches, beans, lentils, soya, strawberries, raspberries, peanuts, melon, cucumber, gooseberries, black currants, marrow squash, pepper, mustard, oranges, lemon, grapefruit, curry, soft margarines, tangerines, other citrus cooking oil (except pure corn oil) and all fruits, grapes, raisins, herbs, including mint, prunes, figs, fruit juices and carbonated drinks including colas.

Latex fruit allergy

A combination unknown to me when I first started out in the 1970s but which has emerged through time is what we call the Latex Fruit Syndrome. A hypersensitivity to latex (raw rubber) is coupled with reactivity to the following foods: almond, apple, apricot, avocado, banana, raw carrot, raw celery, chestnut, cherry, dill, fig, ginger, kiwi, mango, melon, oregano, papaya, passion fruit, peach, pear, plum, raw potato, sage, raw tomato.

If this seems surprising at first, remember that rubber (latex) comes from a plant source: the rubber tree, *Ficus elastica*, which is a kind of fig.

Suspect this and try the necessary exclusions if you know you react to rubber in gloves, elastic, rubber toys, rubber bands, adhesive tape and bandages, condoms etc.

Gluten-free

Sensitivity to gluten, the protein that gives wheat its sticky quality so desired in cooking, was found to be the cause of a serious illness called celiac disease or "sprue." The victim simply wasted away due to malnutrition, while apparently eating normally. The wheat was damaging the gut lining and the body was simply unable to digest and make use of the food being swallowed. These unlucky people must strictly avoid gluten but if they do so, they become quite well.

Gluten sensitivity seems to affect a number of other conditions; for example, *some* cases of multiple sclerosis improve dramatically avoiding it. You might like to try a gluten-free diet, to see if it helps. However, you will need to stick to it for quite some time to be sure (six to eight weeks).

Gluten-free means you must avoid *wheat, oats, barley* and *rye*. Choose flours such as rice, corn, millet and buckwheat instead. Those who have a proven sensitivity to gluten and a real need for gluten-free products are entitled to have them prescribed by their physician.

Doctors place too much reliance on laboratory tests for gluten sensitivity (as usual) and refuse to diagnose it without the characteristic bowel changes. If you feel well avoiding the above four foods then, so far as you are concerned, you have a gluten sensitivity.

Salicylate-free

Salicylic acid (aspirin) and many related compounds can cause allergy reactions, at times very severe. Urticaria and asthma, hyperactivity (in children) and ulcerative colitis are conditions which all the medical fraternity agrees can be caused by salicylate sensitivity.

You might like to try the salicylate-free regime. The foods to avoid are as follows, though the list is not exhaustive:

Fruits
Apples, apricots, pears, oranges, grapefruit, lemon, other citrus fruits, other berry fruits, strawberries, raspberries, pineapples, grapes (raisins), avocadoes, figs, lychees, black and red currants, peaches, guavas, passion fruit, plums (prunes), nectarines, melon, dates, cherries.

Vegetables
Broad and green beans (other pulses OK), watercress, cucumber and other squashes, potatoes (in skins), beets, asparagus, radish, sweet corn, broccoli, carrots, chicory, aubergines (eggplant), tomatoes, spinach, turnips.

Nuts
Almonds, brazils, peanuts, walnuts, macadamia nuts, pine kernels, pistachio nuts, chestnuts and coconuts.

Spices and Herbs (beware!)
Aniseed, cayenne, tarragon, thyme, fenugreek, cinnamon, dill, mace, oregano, paprika, curry, mustard, rosemary, sage, turmeric.

Miscellaneous
Tea, coffee, liquorice, peppermint, cola drinks and honey.

NB: All manufactured foods must be avoided, because of the high incidence of salicylate-type additives.

Yeast-free

Many patients improve on a yeast and mold-free diet. Suspect this especially if you are made ill by alcoholic beverages. For more detail on this, be sure to read chapter 21.

Plan ahead

With most of these additional exclusion steps, it is a good idea to plan ahead. Make sure you have reintroduced enough foods as alternatives that you won't just starve because of the extra restrictions. When you judge there is enough to eat, start the new regime. In general, stick to each trial stage for a minimum of two weeks.

When challenging, follow the same procedure I have described for other foods. But you may sometimes generalize: obviously if three or more salicylate foods react, you would be justified in assuming you have a sensitivity to this compound and not put yourself through more needless reactions; same with the nut-and-pip list.

I would recommend that you fully test each of the gluten foods individually, however. I have seen many people labeled as having "gluten allergy" who were fine eating, say, oats or rye. This was obviously not a true gluten sensitivity but probably wheat allergy.

Fasting

Finally, if all else fails and you have any patience left, you can consider a fast. This will settle once and for all whether there is some other factor in your illness than allergy to food. Review your condition carefully. You have probably been through many trials and tribulations before reaching this point. You might feel like giving up: that is understandable. If you think going on is too difficult, I do urge you to make contact with a professional doctor with skills in this area: generally that means avoid doctors who belong to the American Academy of Allergy Asthma and Immunology (www.aaai. org). They think only in terms of classic allergies, antihistamines and shots. For many years their position papers scoffed at the notion of widespread food allergies.

You should seek a local member of the American Academy of Environmental Medicine (www.aaem.org).

Alternatively, you could opt for the fast.

If you are tired and run down and have lost too much weight, now is not the time to start a fast. Instead, give yourself a break, eat well and take a holiday if you can. Then come back to the problem. A word of warning, however: don't let solicitous busybodies depress you with too many adverse comments. Sometimes this may *make* you feel ill. There is a very powerful psychology at work here. You may be under a great deal of pressure to desist from what you are doing. For one thing, watching others diet makes food addicts feel very uncomfortable, and they may carp at you for what is really no more than a self-centered reason.

Also, there is a tendency to associate weight loss with ill health, though the two are not always connected. Someone, I think rightly, said that we should all weigh the same as we did at the age of twenty-one; few of us do. The so-called 'average weights,' usually quoted from insurance company statistics, include measurement of the obviously obese types. If the upper heavyweights in each height range were excluded as obviously abnormal, then the average weight would fall markedly: in other words, most of us should ideally, weigh less than we do or less than the 'average' weights say we should.

When you are ready to try a fast, the next chapter tells you all you need to know. Eat a full diet for at least two weeks and stoke up with vitamin and mineral supplements in preparation (provided these do not disagree with you).

OTHER REASONS FOR FAILURE

There are other reasons why you may remain ill despite the diet. You may well have food allergies, but there could also be other factors which are denying you your recovery:

Other illnesses concurrent

Sometimes a medical diagnosis is missed: I regularly see patients with an obvious goiter, or abnormal urine tests, anemia and other problems which should have been detected by the family doctor but weren't. If you think this may be the case with yourself, you can go back to your GP and ask about a more thorough check-up. He or she may feel this is unjustified: many doctors view allergy patients as freaks, refusing, regardless of their intelligence or reliability, to take them seriously. In that case you have no option but to ask for a second opinion. It is your right, and your doctor should not be offended by the request.

Chemical sensitivities

These may be to blame in your case, especially if you are well qualified as an 'allergy case' according to the self-inventory. This is quite a complex problem and is the subject of a book at least. It is often necessary to combine a dietary and chemical search in order to draw out the 'eight nails in the shoe.' (page 42)

Thrush infection

It has been found that the causative organism of thrush, *Candida albicans,* is implicated in a wide variety of food and chemical intolerances. Furthermore, it appears to be toxic in its own right. Factors which may suggest the possibility are the following: a known infection (for example, a vaginal irritation that recurs intermittingly); the long-term use of antibiotics for any reason (such as tetracycline for acne); the administration of steroid drugs; the use of the birth control pill for more than two years consecutively; and a tendency to feel worse in damp or moldy conditions or after consuming yeast foods or sugar. If any of these apply to you, see Chapter 21 for more information.

The Human Microbiome

We have gone far beyond the mere "Candida Hypothesis" just referred to; as you will read later, in chapter 21. It's become very exciting.

What we now recognize that healthy bowel flora is more important than keeping unhealthy organisms at bay. The combined pool of trillions of genes from micro-organisms which live in our gut exceed our own meagre supply by a hundred-fold. Genes, you will recall, are what dictate our ability to handle specific proteins.

What has startled scientists is that these micro-flora genes, or the human microbiome, as it's called, also affects our tolerance of foods! So if the gene pool down there in the gut is markedly shifted, so will our food tolerances change. Foods that were once suitable may become toxic to us (and *vice versa*). Dysbiosis, as it's known, is far more serious than we thought.

Malabsorption

It is an unpleasant truth that if you are eating foods which in effect act as poisons you will damage the mucous linings of your intestinal tract. Since these linings are essential for the proper performance of the digestive functions and the selective absorption of necessary vitamins and minerals, most food allergy and intolerance patients become very deficient in proper nutrients. This becomes a self-perpetuating problem because a lack of these nutrients makes the allergy problem worse. Over a long period such deficiencies can become very serious.

We call this condition malabsorption and it is essentially the same problem as celiac disease. Doctors recognize that it occurs with gluten-sensitivity and yet point-blank refuse to accept that it can happen with any other kind of allergy or intolerance.

The whole body depends for its proper functioning on correct and adequate nutrition; therefore it is not surprising if you feel unwell when lacking essential vitamins and minerals. You may need to take extra supplements early on (as a rule we defer this step until you have tracked down all your hidden allergies). Try the effects of taking some basic nutrients. If you experience any improvement, build on this with a much wider supplementation.

Ignore all stupid advice that everything you need is present in a "balanced diet." Even if that were true (it is not), it is of little concern if you are not absorbing properly what you swallow.

Endocrine disorders

Many people feel unwell because of undiagnosed hormonal problems. Many women say they feel worse at period time and, of course, the menopause is a classic time for feeling bad. Most of this is cleared up automatically, once you have sorted out your own best diet. However, it does remain a persistent trouble for some. Occasionally, hormone supplements are the only answer.

Thyroid disease goes undiagnosed even more often. Women with allergies are especially prone to a condition known as auto-immune thyroid disease. This is basically an allergy to her own thyroid gland tissues and extracts. Performance may step up (over-active thyroid) or get worse (under-active). In either event, health is far from optimum.

Treatment for such conditions is outside the scope of this book. You may be able to help your doctor diagnose thyroid insufficiency by keeping a basal temperature chart. Take your temperature every morning before rising, rectally is best, and record the results. If it is consistently below 97.5 (F) or 36.5 (C), this suggests thyroid deficiency. The only really reliable test for auto-immune thyroid disease is an immuno-assay for thyroid antibodies. Discuss it with your doctor.

SUMMARY

If you do not progress while on the elimination diet it is logical to suspect some of the foods you are still eating.

- Did you do the diet correctly in the first place? If not, follow it again without lapses for a further seven days at least.

- If you are then no better, eliminate the 'allowed' foods one at a time for a period of not less than four clear days and test each one on the fifth day, as given in Chapter 12.

- Avoid any food which reacts. Once you start to feel better, also test the original 'banned' foods.

- Try periods of avoiding groups of foods, for example of going meat-free, pulse-free and nut-and-pip-free. If there is any improvement, test each food carefully.

- If all else fails, consider trying a fast. Give yourself a rest and prepare for it by eating plentifully and taking vitamin and mineral supplements.

- Make sure there are no other reasons for feeling unwell. Get another check-up from your doctor, or a second opinion.

14

The Fast: Only if You Must

There are on the market a great many books on the subject of fasting. None of them seem to mention the phenomenon that the food allergy/addiction patient will encounter: withdrawal reactions. Naturally, their authors believe in the health-giving properties of a fast and go on to extol the virtues of a 'good clean-out': *purification* is the ritual word often used. I think a great many readers of these tracts must be severely disappointed and feel misled when they feel bad on a fast – and make no mistake, it is possible to feel dreadful.

Because of the food addictive effect I described in Chapter 7, individuals beginning a fast may experience very unpleasant withdrawal symptoms. Without an understanding of this phenomenon, the response becomes confusing. In many cases, I feel sure, the difficulties may lead to a premature abandonment of the attempt, whereas of course the worse the symptoms due to a fast the more significant the cure – and only persistence brings this.

Moreover, I have seen very little stress laid on the length of time needed for an effective fast. To read some enthusiastic proponents you would imagine that all the benefits are to be had starting the first day, yet this is rarely so. Many even speak of a three-day fast. All this misguided advice is missing the point: it takes about four days to be sure the bowel has cleared, and to fast for a shorter period means you are *not* free of all foods. So you cannot truly tell your response to a fast without persisting at least this many days. Patients with a stubborn bowel may need to allow even longer.

Wasted opportunity

The other common mistake which appalls me because of the wasted opportunity – caused again by a failure to understand the mechanism of allergy and maladaptation – is that sequential reintroduction of foods is never advocated.

If you feel great after a week on a fast, that's *wonderful.* But why? The foolish and ignorant answer is that the deprivation somehow did it. That starving yourself is good for the mind and soul. That's nonsense. Avoiding foods brought the benefits, and the obvious question to anyone quick-witted is: which foods were to blame?

I have heard people say, over and over, they felt outstandingly well on a fast and yet could not tell me one single food they had pinpointed as the reason for the improvement. Most had not even thought of food intolerance or even tried to test individual items. When the fast was deemed over, all normal foods were brought back in, *all at once.* The zealot or writer who introduced them to the idea of fasting had no concept of the elementary science or logic I am sharing with you now. He or she could not see that feeling good on a fast was a clear indicator of one or more foods that made the person ill.

Sometimes the outcome was even sillier: the individual could remember feeling awful quite soon after abandoning the fast – yet had still not made the connection with food allergy and intolerance. He or she was eating those exact foods which had caused the rapid return to everyday unwellness!

Diarrhea and vomiting

You may have never fasted and even consider the idea ridiculous. Yet you may at some time have had a bout of severe gastroenteritis and over the space of a few days had so much diarrhea and vomiting that you emptied your bowel of foods. You may have noticed feeling outstandingly well, despite the preceding days of illness.

Many people have reported this kind of event to me and, again, no one has ever thought of it as a clue to food allergy and intolerance reactions. This is somewhat understandable but nevertheless a wasted opportunity. It is broadcasting exactly the same information as feeling better on a deliberate fast.

Do it properly!

So let me say that the *minimum* fast advocated is four days. That means that if you feel well you can begin introducing foods on the fifth day – *no sooner.* Unless you have a will of iron, you can make it easier on yourself when starting a fast by using a step-down approach. Spend a day eating only a chosen fruit – say, grapes – and drinking spring water. Next day take only the spring water, and you will have moved into a fast fairly effortlessly. Count the grapes-only day as part of the fast, *but only proceed with food testing on the fifth day if you feel quite well.* You would not, of course, test grapes that day in case they are not voided from the bowel.

There is no point in starting the test introductions until you do feel well, so you may need to go on longer than four days. However, without expert medical supervision – and by that I mean a doctor who has had experience of managing fasts – the longest you should continue a fast is for seven days. It has its own hazards, which come into play the longer you carry on; therefore you must not prolong it needlessly.

Let us be quite clear: this is a medical business, not a spiritual process. All we are trying to do is clear the bowel so that we may carry out food tests without the masking effect obscuring the result. The best guide to when your bowel is clear is how you feel. If your symptoms suddenly clear on or about the *fifth* day, that's what we want.

If this has not happened by the eighth morning (unless you have been very constipated), it probably never will and you must desist. In that event it is almost proof positive that you do not have significant food intolerances or allergies and you must look for other explanations for your symptoms instead.

Coping

Responses to fasting vary enormously: some people make light of it and continue their normal work routine. I climbed one of Scotland's highest mountains while on the fourth day of a fast and slept out on the summit under the stars and never felt such vibrant energies, before or since (be sure, I had emergency rations if I had needed sustenance in the wilderness). Others are prostrate and take to their beds for virtually the entire period. Most fall somewhere in between.

You must assume a possible reaction that will prevent you being able to work and make arrangements accordingly. I feel bound to advise you to tell your own doctor what you propose to do in advance. Yet in most cases I am afraid that doing so will invite scorn and hostility, which you must be prepared for. Also, don't expect much helpful advice, because most medical practitioners are simply not trained in this technique; their opinions would rest only on the popular prejudices and misconceptions about food. Having said that, your doctor *is* your doctor, and if you are not prepared to do what he or she says don't go to the office in the first place!

Withdrawal symptoms

It may be worth pointing out that if you should experience withdrawal symptoms, although this can be quite unpleasant, it does point to food addiction and therefore a satisfactory outcome. You may begin to suspect certain foods because of what it is you are craving. You must not give in, of course. But it can be useful to observe, say, a craving for coffee – the feeling that if only you could have a cup, just one cup, you'd feel OK again – it tells you that coffee is almost certainly something you are reacting to.

You may not have suspected it for all those years.

It is astonishing how these effects creep up on us unnoticed. The body gradually learns over time to steer you into taking a "fix" of whatever it needs to settle down. You just think it is something you like. You may even turn to it unconsciously when you meet a stressful situation. But be careful. A tea or coffee craving might really be your body's demand for milk or creamer! A gin and tonic "fix" may really denote a wheat allergy!

Preparation

It is a good idea to prepare for a fast with a few days of good, nutritious eating. For this reason it is not recommended that you fast following a period of severe restrictions on your food intake such as might occur while experimenting with elimination. If that applies to you, return to a full eating program temporarily. This does not mean that junk food must be reintroduced, but simply that you should consume a proper balance of protein, carbohydrates and fat.

The only exception to this advice is when reactions on the elimination diet are so severe that it is easier just to give up eating altogether and slip into a fast for a few days. This usually cuts short the suffering – a process which can be further speeded up by taking Epsom salts, one or two teaspoons in half a glass of warm water, to clear the bowel. Vitamin C (two to ten grams a day) also appears to help, as it often does with toxic reactions. This high dosage should be curtailed as soon as symptoms begin to diminish. Don't wait for a complete recovery, as the vitamin C might itself cause a reaction. This is rare, but if I tell you that most vitamin C is manufactured synthetically from corn derivatives you will see at once why that could apply: Corn is one of the commonest allergens of all.

Avoid chemical exposures during a fast

In my experience, people who are intolerant of foods also have a lot of trouble with chemicals. I have even observed that a chemical exposure can trigger a strong food craving (probably caused by hypoglycemia).

This may not apply to you, but why give yourself an unnecessarily hard time? Don't take risks. It is much more sensible when planning the fast to arrange that you will have as little exposure as possible to any noxious substance. For example, try to avoid urban traffic with its exhaust fumes even if it means staying at home. See to it that no aerosol spray of any kind is used in your presence. Remove perfumes and cosmetics from the bedroom. Do not use powerful detergents, solvents, cleaners or bleach during this period.

Needless to say, you should not smoke during a fast. I repeat again: tobacco is a toxic substance and is almost universally a masked allergy among smokers. Also avoid smoky environments. I have seen smoking a cigarette, or even inhaling second-hand smoke, trigger severe food cravings in sensitive individuals.

Keep away from cats, dogs, dust, pollen and moldy environments if at all possible. If you can't avoid them completely, keep exposure to a minimum.

Paint, especially the gloss type, can be very offensive: make sure you have no contact with freshly decorated rooms. The consequences can take several days to clear up.

Finally, *avoid anything you have found by experience to be inimical to* you. 'Don't court symptoms' is the summary of this section!

I consider it proper to utilize sick leave to carry out a fasting procedure. It is quite legitimate to say you were absent due to illness, because it is in fact true (though it would be better to put your illness on the claim form, rather than write 'fasting,' which is likely to be misunderstood). It is important not to abuse these new privileges, but at the same time you are making a bona fide effort to get well, and – who knows? – in the long run it may result in less absence from work.

It is probably best to avoid contact with strangers where lengthy explanations would be difficult or embarrassing. But your family and friends, who ought to support you, can be the object of a visit or companions for a number of activities; just steer clear of any hostility or scorn.

Constipation

If you find yourself with stubborn constipation on a fast, you may need to consider an enema. It is vital to clear the bowel of all residues, in order to succeed. Sometimes this does not occur spontaneously and you may need mechanical assistance.

Try Epsom salts first, or a gentle infusion of senna pods. If this doesn't work, then arrange an enema. Remember, even if you fasted for as much as three weeks, without adequate bowel movements, it would be useless: not a fast at all, so far as clearing the body is concerned!

How to come off a fast

OK, you have carried out the fast for five days minimum and you feel good. Now you can start re-introducing foods. Instructions for doing this step correctly are even more important than for carrying out the fast itself.

The secret to getting the best outcome is to *begin with foods which are most unlikely to be a problem*. We want to build a platform of safe foods as quickly as possible. Understand this: if you do get a reaction to a test food and it causes symptoms as a result, you will have to wait until the reaction clears up before going on to the next item. While this is not a disaster, it will certainly be most inconvenient: the last thing we want is for you to have to fast for several more days while the symptoms clear!

So we begin with fairly exotic items on the first day. Choose foods you wouldn't normally eat or never have. The table below offers some suggestions, but it is important that you understand you are free to pick your own menu. *Add three new foods a day maximum.* If a food is safe, you may repeat it again as often as you like; so, for example, if salmon is OK you may eat it at every meal along with each new test food until you get bored with it. However, as always, it is better to not be too repetitious – once you have several choices available, make the changes.

After just four days you will have a fallback position of around a dozen safe foods. You won't starve!

From then onwards, test your more usual foods but once again start with those that you consider relatively unlikely troublemakers (meat, fruit and vegetables). Don't risk wheat, milk, coffee, eggs or other 'bogey' foods at this stage, no matter how much you miss them. Try to expand your available diet as far as possible before getting too adventurous.

Finally, of course, you must face up to introducing the probable villains. Remember the reactions can be surprisingly severe. Don't forget to warn your family or friends about this point in advance. If you are unlucky enough to have a bad reaction and – after all, in a way, that's what we are seeking – *continue eating the foods so far found safe.* Take the Epsom salts and bicarbonate mixture described on page 000. Just stop testing new foods until you feel well again; then continue.

Suggested Schedule of Food Tests After a Fast

Days 1– 4		No food
Day 5	Breakfast	Poached salmon
	Lunch	Mango (plus salmon)
	Dinner	Spinach (plus salmon and mango)
Day 6	Breakfast	Baked pheasant, partridge or rabbit (+ salmon, mango, etc.)
	Lunch	Kiwi fruit
	Dinner	Steamed zucchini or squash
Day 7	Breakfast	Lamb chop
	Lunch	Sweet potato
	Dinner	Banana (plus all the above)
and so on.		

If you are doubtful about a particular food, do not try it again for several days, otherwise you may not see a reaction because of the masking effect. Wait five days and then try again. If the second challenge, several days later, is still equivocal, then it is best to treat the food in question as a probable allergen and remove it from the schedule. Do not disregard minor symptoms; these could be significant. Continue only with foods which are demonstrated without doubt to be safe. Incidentally, you may increase the accuracy of these tests by using the pulse check as explained in Chapter 12.

It may happen that without any specific reaction you find yourself unwell again after a number of foods have been reintroduced. Stop as soon as this happens; don't just plough on with more tests. Think back to what you were eating when you were last doing fine and eat only *those* foods till you feel better. Then go on with a different set of new foods. Finally, return to the doubtful ones and sort them out as best you can.

If it still isn't clear which is to blame, abandon them all for ten to twelve weeks and try again. In this way, within ten to fourteen days you should have built yourself a safe diet which you can follow without any untoward symptoms. If so, congratulate yourself: you have done very well. Patience, care and forbearance have brought you their reward: a knowledge of your health that is priceless and could not have been gained any other way.

The half-fast

If you really cannot bear the idea of a total fast, you may follow what I call a half-fast. Simply eat any one fruit and one meat of your choice for the five-day period. Lamb and pears are often chosen, but there is no special magic to them.

All the above advice holds good for the half fast, as for a complete fast, but it goes without saying that you will not get well if you happen to be allergic to either lamb or pears! You must simply take that chance. If you suspect that you may be, simply switch to two other unrelated foods.

The eight-foods diet

Another variation I advocate sometimes is to try eating a small selection of exotic foods; exotic in this context simply means foods you don't normally eat. I usually suggest the patient do this for a longer period, say up to two weeks, before pronouncing it unsuccessful. Eight relatively uncommon foods are selected, and of course spring water. Since this becomes fairly monotonous, you are advised to choose the foods carefully.

A typical choice would be as follows:

Meat	rabbit, turkey
Fruit	kiwis, mango
Vegetables	Rutabaga (swede), spinach
Starch	quinoa, buckwheat

When following this procedure, I always recommend *slow* introductions. Take up to three days with each new food introduced, before you pronounce it safe. As with the fast, foods are added cumulatively. This is very good for children with stubborn eczema.

If the fast doesn't work

In the unlucky event that the fast does not help you, then the probability that you have food allergy and intolerance diminishes close to vanishing point. However, it could be that your illness is compounded of environmental allergies (dust, mold, pollen etc.), chemical sensitivities *and* food allergies. If you eliminate only foods, you may not feel any better because of other exposures unconnected with diet – remember the 'eight nails in the shoe' syndrome? Therefore I still recommend that you follow the schedule of reintroductions as outlined in the previous few sections. You may pick up a surprising reaction from something you didn't suspect.

Of course there may be some other explanation altogether for your symptoms and you are going down the wrong track. I suggest you get help from a good holistic physician.

SUMMARY

1. Eat well before contemplating a fast. The exception is if you have had only one or two days on the exclusion diet and want to switch to a fast.

2. Avoid outside provoking factors on a fast, such as noxious chemicals and stress; yet it is best to stay active if you possibly can.

3. You may go gradually into a fast by having a day on grapes only (or on any other fruit of your choice).

4. If you feel well on Day Five, you may count the grapes day as Day One and start testing any food except grapes. Start by introducing relatively unusual ones so as to avoid the likelihood of a reaction.

5. If you do get a reaction, take a laxative and stop new tests until it clears up. *You may carry on with any foods proved safe up to that point.*

6. If you feel no better due to the fast, your problem is unlikely to be an incompatible food. Nevertheless you may be intolerant of one or more foods, and it is suggested that you follow a reintroduction schedule in order to see if you can spot any that don't agree with you.

15

Controlling Your Diet: How to Stay Well

Success with the Elimination Diet plan may mean that you are restored to health for the first time in many years, or possibly for the first time ever, at least so far as your memory serves.

Staying well is another proposition altogether for some. This isn't meant to be discouraging, and I would like to make it quite clear that the overwhelming majority of people should remain in optimum health provided all that has been set down in these pages is taken to heart and applied in life. Yet I know from experience that some of you are going to have renewed difficulties, and it would be wrong to not try to help with that situation also.

What not to do

I am assuming that you carried out all the procedures correctly, felt better and continued to avoid those foods which demonstrably made you ill. If your deterioration took place quite soon after reintroducing 'safe' foods, then the chances are that one or more items have slipped through the net and back into your eating pattern which shouldn't have. Return to the full elimination diet and see if that corrects it; if it does, then re-test foods slowly and more thoroughly. The rest of this chapter may not necessarily apply to you.

Self control

If you began eating 'forbidden foods' once again because of cravings and your symptoms returned, then I think you know what to do. All you need is will-power – or common sense, whichever you are shortest on!

I have been astonished over the years by how quickly some patients would lapse. For many I think it was a state of denial: he or she simply did not *want* to accept that their favorite foods made them seriously ill. One consultant physician in my home city – who did well to swallow his pride and come to me – I found reacted badly to apples. He ate several each day and this is what caused the majority of his symptoms. We laughed over the irony of the saying "An apple a day keeps the doctor away"; not in his case! There were one or two lesser reactions as I recall. He went away very happy to be rid of his problems.

I was surprised when only a few weeks later he rang me and said his symptoms had come back. I asked him the question I ask every single patient in this situation: "Have you stayed off the allergy food completely?" He admitted he was back to eating apples, one or two a day. It was hard not to be derisive but I did my best to control my disposition and gently pointed out that this was why the symptoms had returned. My colleague hemmed and hawed and really just could not bring himself to admit that might be the reason his symptoms had returned.

I finally got his understanding that he must stay off apples for a year or more and then have only one every few days, never more. Only then, providing his symptoms did not return.

If this description fits your situation, you need to get a grip and realize that you are being punished by Nature for being so foolish. She is kind enough to give you symptoms as a clear message that you should NOT eat the food. You will ignore this sign at your peril.

New allergies

However, if you have been conscientious and carefully continued an eating program which was successful at first but now seems to be leading inexorably back to illness, you must look for a reason.

It happens, so don't feel negative about yourself or the diet.

The likelihood is that you are developing new intolerance reactions to those foods which were safe at first. To understand how this can happen you will recall that earlier I pointed out that the frequent consumption of a food increases its adverse potential.

The rules of adaptation will apply, and although at first your body may be quite able to tolerate this exposure it is possible that maladaptation will gradually develop from excessive use of a food.

In this case you will be forced to give the food a rest and look for other alternatives. If it appears to be a recurring problem, there is little choice but to adopt a rotation diet, which is described next.

New intolerances for old

One of the most daunting problems confronting me over the years was the patient who constantly develops new food reactions: no sooner have a number of 'safe' foods been found than those also start to cause symptoms. Certain individuals trying to work out their own allergies – and you may be such a one –will also encounter this nuisance and be frustrated by it. Fortunately it isn't a very common occurrence, except among severely ill patients, but it is important to know how to deal with it when it happens.

The answer was evolved in the 1930s by Dr Herbert Rinkel, a perceptive and clever American allergist, one of the real founders of clinical ecology as a science. It is the *rotary diversified diet*. Do not confuse this with the popular "rotation diet" published in the 1980s by Martin Katahn, which showed little of the understanding I am sharing here [Martin Katahn, *The Rotation Diet: lose up to a pound a day and never gain it back*, Bantam Books, New York, 1987]

In principle the real rotation diet isn't very hard to understand. It simply requires that each individual food, instead of being eaten at random, is taken according to a precise timetable. There are no 'daily' foods. Once eaten, a particular item is not then repeated for a set interval, which may be four, five or seven days. Instead it is 'rotated' with other foods, themselves eaten at fixed intervals also.

To make this clearer, take beef as an example. It may be eaten on, say, Monday and then not again until the following Friday (a four-day rotation). Pork, on the other hand, may be eaten on Tuesday but then not again until Saturday, and so on.

This considerably eases the load of allergens or *potential* allergens to which the body is being subjected. If there is less exposure to any one food, there is less likelihood of it reacting. Thus this type of diet is quite therapeutic: poorly tolerated or marginal reactors may become instead very minimal and non-reacting respectively. It will also reduce the chances of new allergies developing. This could be very important to people who can find few non-allergic foods. Unfortunately, these are precisely the individuals who are likely to become quickly allergic to other substances. Theirs is a difficult problem, and a rotation diet is really quite vital.

There is also a third advantage: a proper rotation diet may be diagnostic, in other words it enables one to identify reacting foods. Substances are eaten infrequently deliberately, so that *the masking effect will not work*. The key to this is allowing the body to become clear of that food before eating it again; thus previously hidden allergies will expose themselves, or if a new reaction should somehow develop it will at least declare itself and become obvious. It will not be able to make you critically ill; you will know, and all you will have to do is drop it from the rotation plan, replacing it with a new food that you have found safe on testing.

I like to point out that Nature rotates our foods for us – or it happened in the past. As the seasons passed through their changes, first one crop then another became available. Spring vegetables would fade and be replaced by those of summer, fall and winter. Fruits would come in due season, last a few weeks, and then vanish.

Ingenuity enabled Man to harvest and store some foods, against cold winters or leaner times. But storage was not entirely safe; foods would loose nutrients. This often meant that by the end of winter, most foods were depleted of essential vitamins and if you take the trouble to look at historical accounts (I have) you will see that *spring was often the danger time*, when people would weaken and die of malnutrition. Scurvy was rife. The problem paradoxically occurred in the midst of spring's abundance; it marked the end of winter's long nutritional deprivation, before the new crops could grow.

In fact I am willing to speculate that this is one of the reasons that most of the early great civilizations sprang up in warmer climes: that the annual winter cull of weaker humans did not take place because of the availability of foods all year round.

Once farming had moved beyond the Medieval feudal system to commercial market-oriented gardening, foods were grown and moved around according to available markets. This meant that cold snowy Northern Europe could feed itself and the stage was set for the greatest of all civilizations to evolve.

Constructing a rotation diet

It isn't difficult to design a rotation diet, given certain basic rules, and patients should learn to do it for themselves; after all, no one else is in such a good position to understand his or her own likes and dislikes. True, some selections have to be made for scientific reasons, but there is always scope for culinary and gastronomic preferences. A rotation diet is essentially a personalized thing: what works well for one person may not suit another (or even keep him or her healthy).

However, one very important piece of information you need before tackling one for yourself is an understanding of "food families." These are groups of plants and animals that are related chemically in such a way that the body treats them as being similar from the metabolic point of view; in other words, if you react to one member of a group you are quite likely (but not absolutely certain) to react to others of the same family. It is perhaps obvious to you that cabbage, cauliflower and Brussels sprouts are related, but it may not be quite so obvious that mustard, turnips and rutabaga (swede) are also in that same group, which also includes beet greens, bok choy, broccoli, Chinese cabbage, collard greens, garden cress, horseradish, kale, kohlrabi, mustard greens, radishes, sea kale, swiss chard and turnip greens. We call this group of foods the *Brassicas;* formerly it was known as the *Crucifer* family and sometimes still appears in lists under that name. There are over 3,000 species of mustard alone. Rape (as rapeseed) and canola are less well-known members of this very large and commercially important *food family.* (Wikipedia on-line)

Similarly, carrots, parsnips, celery and parsley belong to the same family (one of my child patients pointed out how similar the green frond tops are). Tobacco, potato, tomato, aubergine and pepper may seem an even less likely set, but they are in fact all in the *nightshade* family, named after the deadly nightshade plant, *Atropa belladonna* (very poisonous, hence its popular name). Grains, of course, go together. Wheat seems to be the worst offender, followed by corn and the others not far behind. You have read my condemnation of this group of foods in several places in this book. Collectively, they cause more problems than any other – and they are taken collectively because they *are* a family. (Incidentally, sugar cane is also a member; these are all *grasses* of some kind.)

Why are food families important at this stage?

Because, as well as making sure that any single food does not occur too often, you must also take some care that foods from the same family do not come close together too frequently.

To help you in this a comprehensive list of food families is provided in appendix A. You must refer to it when working out your scheme. In general, we allow members of the same family to be taken at an interval of two days, even when specific foods are rotated one day in four. This supposes that no other member of the same group is eaten between the two. In other words, wheat on Monday, oats on Wednesday is fine; then wheat again on Friday (or barley or rice but not oats).

So you will see that knowledge of the food families is really quite essential to the construction of a proper rotation diet. It is, of course, possible to eat more than one food a day! The simplest regimen allows you to eat a given food (or food family) several times on the permitted day. To give you an idea of how this works I have constructed a simple table based on this principle:

Food	*Day 1*	*Day 2*	*Day 3*	*Day 4*
Meat	beef	pork	lamb	chicken
Fruit	pears or apples	grapes	banana	orange
Vegetables	peas or beans	cauliflower cabbage	celery carrot	tomato lettuce
Cereal/starch	wheat	buckwheat	rice	potato
Drink	apple juice	grape juice	pineapple juice	orange juice
Miscellaneous	milk	raisins	nuts	egg

The left-hand column gives pointers to the kind of food chosen. There is a meat for each day, a vegetable, a fruit and so on. The table is read *vertically*: for example, on Day I you may eat beef, apple, pear, peas, beans, wheat and drink apple juice or milk. Milk is placed on the same day as beef since it comes from the same animal; similarly chicken and egg.

It may be possible, if the intolerance is mild, to rotate one grain food each day (wheat, barley, rice, oats perhaps). Otherwise, you must conform to the rules with regard to the starches or 'filler' row, as written.

One or two other points are worth commenting on. Potato is not, of course a cereal, but it is a great substitute. Patients like a 'filler' food, something that satisfies. Potato does this just as well as bread or oatmeal. Potato flour is available commercially and can be used in the same way as ordinary flour, though it doesn't behave in the same manner when used for cooking.

If we were allergic to cow's milk, soya milk might be an acceptable substitute. Of course, it must only be drunk on Day One, along with peas and beans, also members of the family of *legumes* or *pulses*. Furthermore, most soya milk preparations contain cane sugar, thus you would not be able to eat this substance on any other day.

You will see that fruit juice from the appropriate source is used to drink each day. In *addition* to this you could take a herb tea. Spring water is acceptable at any time.

Avoid incompatible foods

It is important to stress that you should not include foods to which you know you are intolerant. It is better to avoid these for a few months and then test them in accordance with the instructions given in Chapter 12. If at that time there is no reaction, you may then include that food in the rotation scheme, making due allowance for food families.

Try to get organic foods if you can. Manufactured items are not permitted because of adulteration; for example, a beef-burger may contain not only beef, but soya, wheat (rusk), onion and several other items which cut right across the rotation plan. Similarly, complex foods, such as cake, are not allowed. You must eat only simple unprocessed items, bought fresh. This in itself makes for an improvement in health.

> Advice on how to considerably reduce your exposure to pesticides in food comes from the Environmental Working Group. They maintain that if you avoid the "dirty dozen" pesticide contaminated fruits and vegetables you can reduce your pesticide exposure by over 90%. Their currently published lists of "clean" and "dirty" foods are given in appendix D.

Once you have worked out a successful rotation diet on which you feel well, it should continue to support you in good health, perhaps indefinitely, barring any adversity or stress. That means many of your formerly allergic foods can be avoided for long periods; thus you may lose many food allergies by regaining your tolerance.

Eventually, you should be able to enjoy, in moderation, many of your favorite indulgences. However, it must be stressed that these must only be returned to your diet on a rotation basis, otherwise you will soon be in trouble with them again. Remember: you may lose your individual allergies, but you are unlikely to lose the tendency to develop them.

The best long-term answer to allergy and intolerance is overall wellness, meaning: develop a healthy lifestyle, healthy relationships, a healthy work environment and nourishing personal answers to the meaning of life. Identify your goals and harmonize them with what you are doing, your lifetime values and the goals and values of others around you.

General well being, I have found, is the best "cure" for allergy and intolerance problems. Avoidance and control of allergies and intolerance, as described in this and other chapters in the book, should really only be a short-term solution, while your body recovers its balance.

However that's altogether another book (which I'm planning!)

Extending the rotation diet

The above diet is fairly simple and can be extended in a number of ways: for example you may add a nut each day, a hot drink, a cold drink, a fish and so on. The only practical limits on this are just how much complexity you can allow without getting confused and making mistakes and how many safe foods you can find. Keep food families firmly in mind when making an addition, and don't cross these; in general, add similar foods on the same day. Nevertheless, you may find you are able to tolerate members of the same family on alternate days: to some extent this is a case of trial and error.

A more elaborate rotation diet is given below, to give you an idea of what can be done with a bit of ingenuity. It may save you the bother of making up your own.

This is the province of unusual and very sick patients. The average reader would do well to skip the remainder of this chapter, which I have included as a duty to those who need extra help and are without a knowledgeable healthcare specialist.

Day	1	2	3	4
Meat	Pork	Beef	Lamb	Rabbit
Fowl	Chicken	Turkey	Pheasant	Duck
Fish	Cod Pollock	Salmon Trout	Halibut Flounder	Mackerel Tuna
Vegetables	Peas Fava bean Carrot Cabbage Cauliflower	Potato Peppers Leek Butternut squash Artichoke	Lentil Green beans Parsnip Broccoli Celery	Tomato Lettuce Onion Zucchini Asparagus
Fruit	Apple Banana Strawberry Kiwi	Orange Grape (raisin) Melon Peach	Pear Pineapple Raspberry Papaya	Grapefruit Raisins Mango Nectarine
Starch	Wheat Corn	Buckwheat Sago	Rice Oats	Tapioca Quinoa
Drinks	Chamomile tea Apple juice	Fennel tea Grape juice	Rooibos Pineapple juice	Rosehip Grapefruit juice
Nuts	Brazil	Cashew	Walnut	Hazelnuts
Cooking oil	Corn	Olive	Peanuts	Sunflower
Specials	Yams Scallops Soya milk Chocolate	Dates Shrimps Milk Honey	Sweet potato Venison Coffee Carob	Figs Lobster Goat's milk

More severe cases

Unfortunately, this straightforward approach may not be enough. Some people – again, usually the severe cases – need to follow a stricter set of rules in relation to rotating in order to be successful. How do you know if this applies to you? Well, it's fairly simple: if you felt well for a week or two on the elimination diet and then your symptoms returned, and then the same thing happened with a simple rotation diet, you must place yourself in the category of those quick to develop new food reactions. In effect, you are an extremely sensitive person, intolerant of foods and, by inference, of chemicals also.

Your task will be to work out a rotation diet based on the principle of 'One food, one meal.' This may sound drastically restrictive, and in fact it is; but in almost all situations it is better than feeling ill. It will keep you fairly skinny – but if you feel well again, do you really care? Besides, if you have followed the book so far and understand about food addiction you will realize that being plump or 'meaty' is far from being healthy. This is especially true of babies, where round, chubby features and a ruddy glow are so much admired. It is a totally false standard of health.

No one wants you to be emaciated, but there is a happy weight for you which is doubtless lower than your friends think it should be. Don't let them worry you with ignorant concern.

I've prepared below a sample of this kind of diet. This time it is rotated through four days. Spring water is permitted at any time. Moreover, you may be able to tolerate one cup of herb tea, but this must also be rotated (there are many varieties to choose from).

Paste a copy of your final workable diet on the door to the refrigerator, or somewhere in the kitchen, to serve as a reminder. It is surprising how quickly you learn it by heart.

Problems with the rotation diet

It is possible for your tolerance of a food to break down, even on a rotation diet. This could be caused by extra stress or an acute illness, or by exposure to some other type of toxin, such as a gas leak or chemical spraying. It is unfortunate if this happens, but very important that you know how to deal with it. The key to this is planning ahead. As soon as you succeed in making the rotation diet work for you – that is, as soon as your symptoms subside and stay that way – at once begin testing to identify new and useful foods. Don't wait until the problem arrives before solving it; be ready.

After a week on the diet, *all other foods are now unmasked.* You can test one or two, following the usual procedure. Any that you find safe can be held in reserve in case you need them. You don't need many, especially if you pick items from rare families that will fit more or less anywhere into the rotation without cutting across the scheme. Don't spend too much time experimenting if it makes you ill; concentrate on maintaining your well-being instead. Just do this step before you need to. If a food does start to cause a reaction, you will then be able to substitute it at once.

The following examples are foods which are to all intents and purposes separate families in their own right: eel, horsemeat, pigeon, carp, guava, brazil nut, macadamia nut, papaya, pineapple, persimmon, kiwi fruit (Chinese gooseberry), sweet potato, sesame and yam. Not all of them are easily available unless you happen to live in a large cosmopolitan city, with multiracial groups and shops; but the principle is important. By consulting the more extensive list of food families given in appendix A you should be able to choose items that are not related to foods that you personally were accustomed to eating.

As the weeks and months go by, you will be 'resting' quite a lot of foods and should recover your tolerance of many of these. At this stage it is worth testing and introducing some foods solely for the sake of variety. You can begin eating new substances and give old ones a rest. This way, although you may only eat twenty-one foods in a week, you could be cycling through a 'repertoire' of twice that number.

The only limit is how many you can keep track of without becoming confused; naturally, you should try to avoid mistakes. If it does become necessary to omit a food which was formerly safe, wait about three months and try again. If it no longer reacts, re-include it in the rotation if you wish. If it still causes symptoms, leave it for a further six months and then try again.

Extreme cases

The other great problem you will encounter on making this diet work for you is the question of organic foods. If you are so exquisitely sensitive that you need the diet, then it is almost certain you will be unable to cope with the chemical adulteration of food produce: vegetables are sprayed; fruits waxed or, when dried, bleached and oiled; animals force-fed on fattening chemicals and poultry treated with hormones. Then there is the problem of packaging and shipment: bananas are treated with ethylene, meats wrapped in polythene and juices put in cartons waterproofed with a corn derivative, to give just a few examples.

The problem is really quite a complex one. There do seem to be people who react to almost everything in their environment. Théron Randolph calls them 'universal reactors.' This is a distressing state to be in: it really does seem to be the case that the world they live in is too hostile to cope with. 'Total allergy syndrome' is a dramatic-sounding journalistic phrase to describe this unfortunate affliction (a term never used by doctors), and you may read bizarre stories about it in the popular press. I find these cases reported rather regrettable: it is important that the public do not form an impression of allergy sufferers as freaks and crackpots, which is how these wretched sufferers are often portrayed. My personal campaign has been to educate the public to the view that allergies are not only 'normal' but very common.

If you are among those who are made ill by so many factors that they cannot escape from enough of them in order to feel any better, it is pretty hopeless trying to go it alone. It would be far better for you to contact a skilled physician through the American Academy of Environmental Illness (www.aaei.com).

16

Children as Special Patients

Children and their diets

Imagine being completely unable to help yourself and relying on others for your welfare. Suppose those in charge of you pumped you full of noxious foods that poisoned you (in effect) and made you feel sickly, irritable, fretful and dazed. Then they blamed *you* for misbehaving and being 'naughty' when all the time you were unable even to think straight. You tried to refuse some of these foods but were made to eat them because those who controlled you insisted mistakenly that you *must* eat them because they were 'good for you.' You would get pretty fed up with this state of affairs, wouldn't you?

Well, of course you would; yet this is the lot of many children with food allergies and intolerance. A large number of children are made to eat things they would be better not to because of ignorance or myths concerning the value of certain foods.

One of the common errors is that milk is necessary for calcium for bones and teeth. This is nothing more than propaganda of the milk marketing authorities, aided and abetted by ignorant doctors and foolish dieticians. The truth is that, far from being essential, it is one of the most pernicious foods known, and many people avoid it all their lives and only feel ill if they take it.

Another fallacy is that sugar provides energy: in fact, it saps it faster than any substance you can eat – it only *appears* to give energy because it creates the lethargic feeling in the first place. There are many others which I need not list here. And all the while cunning advertising sales campaigns are busy daily adding falsehoods and misinformation to the confusing pile of 'facts,' and the poor, besieged housewife has to cope with in trying to feed her family well.

A child's preferences, if you will allow them, *may* be a guide to you. A strong aversion to a particular food may be nature's way of pointing out that it is an incompatible food, thus parents should *never* force their children to eat foods they dislike. Yet the other side of the same coin is that once food addictions have become established, then the child's 'preference' is really only a craving for a food. So when it comes to the diet I usually advise parents to tell the child that he or she may *not* eat the banned foods but is not *compelled* to eat the allowed ones.

This puts hunger on your side: the child either eats the right food or goes without. After a day or two of sulking and getting over the withdrawals, the child will invariably co-operate; yet he or she has the option of avoiding foods that are deeply and instinctively disliked. The difficulty I always find during this period of laying down the rules lies with the parents: to many of them it seems downright heartless to be so unyielding on the subject of what their youngster may or may not eat. I only ask them to try, and in most cases it works very well.

The fact is a lot of children are picky eaters because of their addiction to the wrong foods. Parents sometimes complain that their child already eats very little, so further restrictions mean that they may not eat at all. I explain that this pickiness is really due to the fact that the child is being poisoned by what he or she is already eating. As soon as the bowel clears of these harmful substances, the child's appetite always returns and little Johnny will often show an astonishing gusto for eating, where before he showed only apathy and indifference to food. In the meantime, the previous paragraph applies. *If the child does not eat on this plan, he or she will get well nevertheless. It is vital to understand this is about exclusions.*

Does your child have food incompatibilities?

The self-inventory in Chapter 10 will provide you with many clues that may make it obvious that your child has allergies. Nevertheless, many of the symptoms are very subjective: you wouldn't know if your child were experiencing many of them. Accordingly, I have supplied below a table of objective signs and observations that may help you to decide. Once again, it should be pointed out that the symptoms may have other causes, but the more of those below that are positive, the more certain it is that the child's problem is an allergy or genetic food incompatibility:

Picky eater	Irritability
So-called 'growing pains'	Convulsions, fits
Abnormal temper tantrums	Blackouts
Moodiness or crying	'Blank spells'
Always on the go, very active	Destructive, smashing up attacks
Mood swings, high to low and back	Excitement or silliness
Very pale	Dark rings under the eyes
Runny nose	Puffy face, swollen eyes
Prolonged bed wetting	Melancholic, inconsolable
Recurring sore throats	Recurring ear infections
Recurring bouts of abdominal pain	The "allergic salute"
Failure to thrive or mantain weight	Poor sleep, sleep apnea

Children suffer from food allergies just as adults do, and some have a very hard time of it. The typical victim would be fussy with his or her food, eat poorly, have frequent coughs and colds, sleep badly and seem endlessly naughty. "Allergic shiners" may be evidence: dark black rings around the eyes, set in a pallid face. The "allergic salute," if you have not heard of it, is a child pushing up his or her nose with the flat of the hand, usually accompanied by sniffing, in an effort to keep back the mucus. This may be so persistent that the child develops a crease across the bridge of the nose.

Skin rashes are very common; so are sore throats and ear infections. Many children end up having their tonsils and adenoids out in a desperate attempt to tackle the problem of recurring infections, and all the while unsuspected, it is something in the diet which is the cause of the immune compromise.

Incidentally, this may be the place to remark that the relative frequency of allergy foods for children seems to differ somewhat from the adult table of offenders. For grown-ups the 'top of the league' is wheat. Dairy comes second, followed by tea and coffee. But for children there is no contest: the number one offender is milk. This is followed by colorings and chemicals, such as glutamates, corn (as high fructose corn syrup mainly), and then wheat.

Elimination dieting for children

Youngsters may pose special problems when it comes to elimination dieting. In some ways they are better able to tolerate special diets than adults. Perhaps this is part of a child's conditioning to do as he or she is told – I don't know. Certainly many of my young patients are extraordinarily understanding about their condition. When offered something to eat which is not permitted, they will refuse politely and explain why, sometimes to the chagrin of the offending adult! We should credit them with a sensible basic nature and an intelligent desire not to be ill. Who wants to feel ill? Adults don't, so why should children?

On the other hand, the opposite is sometimes true. A youngster may have a very trying time on the elimination diet. Probably he or she does not understand the explanations given, and since he or she cannot see the reason for the restrictions, does not co-operate. These are among the most difficult cases of all, because the truth is that if children want to cheat it is always possible for them to do so. One young boy I know was accustomed to sneaking out of bed at three in the morning and emptying the sugar bowl while his parents slept. His mother said she had noticed the family seemed to be consuming a great deal of sugar but never caught on to what was happening until she awoke with a headache one night, got up for an aspirin and caught the miscreant in the act.

The children who fall into this latter category actually need much more support and solicitude. It is tempting to admonish him or her for being 'naughty,' but really it should be remembered that the withdrawal symptoms can be quite distressing and that scolding will only lower the child's spirits still further. It's a tough diet for an adult who is well motivated, so it is certainly tough for a child. Encouragement is what is needed – admiration even.

Easing the pain!

For children, I would make certain exceptions to the test diet regime, to make it easier for the young heart and mind to cope with the restrictions.

I would generally allow rice cakes. Rice is a relatively uncommon grain allergy, especially in non-Asians. Dairy-free margarine can be permitted but make sure it is wheat-free: yes, wheat occurs sometimes in "alternative" margarines. Note that I would not be concerned about the presence of trans-fats in a situation like this. Short-term exposure to unsuitable nutrients of this sort poses little or no danger. Arterial damage accrues from years or even decades of faulty food consumption, not just a few days.

In this situation, the major advantages to be gained from avoiding deadly foods far outweighs the minor risk – a demographic risk at that – from consuming suspect alternatives, *provided the substitute was clean, wholesome and did not contain stray residues of banned foods.*

I would also permit honey, in small quantities. I emphasize *small*. Honey is just another sugar food. Qualitatively, it has nothing much to recommend it over refined sugar and is not as good as raw sugar. But sugar, usually from the cane plant, is from the grass family and so most unsuitable. Honey, by empirical experience, I found to be little trouble.

By permitting honey in small quantities, it was possible to gear up to certain "treats" that were healthy and persuasive substitutes for candy, sodas and confections. I will be offering a few simple recipes in a later chapter for honeyed-treats, such as banana surprise, carob brownies and peanut butter squares. The psychological value of such rewards, judiciously used, could have a very beneficial effect on the young patient.

For the same reason, sugar-free jams were allowed. The French brand *Bonne Maman* was good and I see it is available in the USA today. There are plenty of others to track down; just avoid the dishonest brands which sell "sugar-free" jam, meaning it has corn syrup as a sweetener. Strictly speaking, these products would all be considered manufactured. But a good natural jam is made only with the fruit and not with sugar. Of course, without the sugar, there is no preservative quality and such conserves must be kept in the refrigerator, otherwise they go moldy. But for the child's delight and, considering the remote risk of a reaction, I found it a worthwhile compromise.

If the child is on a salicylate-free (p. 145) or nut-and-pip free diet (p. 143), then obviously fruit jams cannot be permitted.

Some treats for kids (and grown ups)

Here are a few delicious treats that are safe for youngsters. You'll have all the kids at school queuing up to dip into your child's lunch box!

I have already indicated that I allow a little leeway for kids. But I know that adults find these treats great too and can enjoy them, knowing they are (in the main) safe alternatives to the usual candies and confections.

Peanut butter squares
(wheat-free, egg-free, dairy free if you want)

- 4 tbsps pure peanut butter (no additives)
- 4 tbsps non-set (runny) honey
- 1/3 cup (2 oz) sesame seed (or lightly blended nuts)
- 1/3 cup (2 oz) dried coconut
- 1/3 cup (2 oz) dried goat's milk powder (could be gram flour or soya flour)

Melt the honey gently, stir in the peanut butter and other ingredients until well mixed. If too stiff to work, add a little olive oil. Spread out in a flat tin and slice into squares. When set, separate the pieces like candy. Tip: pop the tray in the fridge to speed up setting.

These won't last long!

Carob brownies (chocolate substitute)
(wheat-free, dairy-free)

- 3 tbsps oil
- ½ cup (3 oz) of soya flour, gram flour (garbanzo) or ground sunflower seeds
- 2-3 tbsps honey
- 2 eggs beaten (once you know they are safe) otherwise see egg replacer suggestions on page 000.
- 2 tsp baking powder
- 1/3 cup (2 ozs) carob powder
- 1 tsp vanilla essence (extract)
- 1/3 cup (2 ozs) chopped walnuts or pecans
- pinch of salt

Melt the oil and honey over a low heat, then cool. Add cocoa or carob powder and mix well. Beat in the eggs or replacer. Stir in flour, baking powder, salt, vanilla extract and nuts. Add water as needed to keep the mixture moving.

Put heaped teaspoons into muffin tins (for 12-16 brownies) and bake in the center of the oven at 325⁰ for 20- 30 minutes. Tip: test any cake by sticking a toothpick or clean knife into the center. If it comes out clean, they are done.

Banana treat
(wheat-free, dairy-free, egg-free, sugar-free)

- Take a medium to large banana and slice in two lengthways.
- Spread pure peanut butter (no additives) in between the slices, sandwich-style. Put the top strip back on, drizzle over with (pure) honey and sprinkle with sesame seeds, which stick nicely to the honey.

Delicious and all natural. Limit of one a day!

Sweet potato pudding

Peel sweet potatoes and grate them, so you have about 1 cupful per person.

Put in a pan and just cover with soya milk. Add maple syrup, 1 tsp per person, and a little ground nutmeg. Cook in a hot oven till soft and mushy, about 20 minutes at 375F/190C.

Carrot cake
(wheat-free, dairy-free, egg-free, sugar-free)

- 1 medium carrot, grated
- 2 heaped tbsps any allowed non-grain flour (alternatively, fine grind some almonds)
- 2 heaped tbsps currants, or raisins softened by soaking
- ½ tbsp oil (use more to get the right consistency)
- ¼ tsp cinnamon powder
- 1 tsp honey

Combine all ingredients together and mix well. Press the moist mixture into a greased and lined 4-inch (10cm.) cake tin and bake in the oven at 375⁰ F/190⁰C, for 25 minutes.

This keeps moist for up to 4 days.

Better than fries

Commercial fries are out. They are treated with MSG and sugar is added. Kids, we know, love fries. Here is a healthy and tasty replacer:

Quick and tasty coconut "spuds" (potatoes)

Ingredients:
1 large baking potato per person (preferably organic)
1 clove garlic per person (preferably organic)
1 dessertspoon of organic virgin coconut oil per person

Preheat oven to 395F/200° C. Melt the coconut oil in the oven in a large baking dish. Peel and thickly slice the potatoes and the garlic and place them in the dish, making sure they are well covered with the melted coconut oil. Sprinkle to taste with organic sea salt. Check them after 20 minutes and turn. Cook for a 20 minutes more, or until crunchy (and very yummy!)

You can also make fries with sweet potato (Spanish *batata*); just cut them into penny slices and fry lightly till golden brown. You can make a sweet potato jacket by baking it, slitting it open, drizzling coconut oil inside and dusting with powdered cinnamon or ground nutmeg.

Challenge testing for childen

Children are surprisingly tolerant of diet testing. Their natural curiosity helps them participate in the investigations.

The same holds true for challenge testing. A child who has suffered unpleasant symptoms as a result of eating a food will usually not crave it any further, so challenge tests can be very helpful. Nobody likes to feel ill or different and once the child understands where the problem is coming from, he or she will be extremely co-operative in ongoing exclusions. How unlike many adults who do not behave intelligently, even when compelling evidence of incompatible foods and the damage they cause is staring them in the face.

Sharing the burden

It will certainly help if the grown-ups and siblings can join in on the diet and I usually recommend this. For one thing, this will give the rest of the family a vivid idea of what it takes to go through with the program. Also – and this is quite an important point – it will help the child not to feel different or peculiar.

There is one other practical reason why families should join in. From what you have read you will realize that it is most unlikely that a child with allergies is the only one in the family to have them. After all, he or she only eats what is offered; if the child's diet is faulty, then so is that of the rest of the family.

The probability is that the mother or father also has the problem, perhaps without realizing it. But there is only one way for parents to find out for sure, and that is to try the *Diet Wise* plan for themselves.

Almost everyone feels better on the elimination diet once the withdrawal phase is over, so it is worth a try.

Mothers can be difficult I have found. There is an image of motherhood, beloved by all, in which she is a fountain of 'goodies' such as cake, sweets, cookies and delicious puddings. Children, sadly, may judge her love for them purely in terms of this rather artificial archetype. It is all very well in the pages of Enid Blyton or in the land of hobbits, but in real life such outpourings from the kitchen can be deadly: Yes, deadly. Countless husbands die early because of a wife's well-meaning ignorance in the kitchen.

Thus mothers (and fathers too) may try to be 'kind' to the youngster by allowing sweets and other forbidden treats on the diet. Of course, in the long term this is hardly being kind; it is downright irresponsible and may rob the child of his or her rightful recovery. It is simply not possible to cheat 'slightly' on this program and expect results. We are trying to *clear the bowel,* and this cannot be achieved unless the regime is adhered to strictly.

Neighbors and relatives can be obstructive for the same misguided reasons. Not understanding what it is that you are trying to do, they may feel the child is being deprived and reason that it is perfectly all right to defy your wishes in this matter. My advice is that unless you can be quite certain of cooperation you should keep the youngster away from the care of family and others for the period in question. It is only a week or two, and this should pose no strain on family relationships.

Games and rewards

There is no doubt at all that the best way to ensure the cooperation of children is to induce them to follow the diet on the strength of their own decision to do so. One of the best ways to do this is to make it into a game. If there are rewards for eating properly, commensurate with their idea of the effort involved, it will usually be a success. There are as many ways to do this as there are children, but it is a good idea to have rewards on a day-to-day basis, since the attention span of youngsters is notoriously short.

This can be followed up by a larger prize for achieving a whole week of successes. The old black marks and stars idea is good for many more miles yet. There could be stars for each successful day and a gold star for the week. Black marks would, needless to say, go unrewarded and would jeopardize the weekly score, which should be punishment enough in itself.

This is far more satisfactory than the use of force or punishment to ensure compliance, which smothers initiative; besides, the child may reason that the diet is worse than any punishment you might inflict, in which case you cannot hope to succeed! But a much more important point is that he or she will have enough to cope with that is unpleasant, at least for the first few days, without your adding disciplinary actions to the misery. Have confidence in your child: it is amazing the number of frightful, disobedient monsters that settle down and become placid and sociable after a few days without junk food and sugar pep.

You could be in for a pleasant surprise, but you will never know unless you loosen the reins a little.

It might seem silly to point it out, but perhaps it needs saying: sweets and other diet items should not form part of a reward system. Try to cultivate the point of view that they are harmful, not something kind parents give out. Thus don't be tempted into making sweets the *big* reward when it is all over – that encourages the wrong attitude. You want the child to completely change his or her thinking, permanently, not just 'until it's all over.' You see, the chances will be quite high of having to go on avoiding certain foods if the child is to remain healthy, so in that sense it will never be 'all over.' Perhaps you need to revise your own thinking on the topic, too.

School meals

It is definitely easier to manage the diet of pre-school youngsters than that of older children: at home you at least have a fighting chance of controlling what they eat. School meals are particularly disastrous and must be avoided at all costs. It is sometimes possible to secure the help of a teacher in supervising what the child eats, but make sure this is someone you can depend on or you may face ridicule for your ideas and possibly open contempt of your requests. Unfortunately, there is a general misconception among teachers that, because they are held liable for the safe custody of a child at school, the parents' wishes don't count for a thing when it comes to the child's management.

It is undoubtedly best if you can bring your child home for meals at lunchtime. If this is impossible, the options are to provide a packed lunch within the guidelines of the elimination diet or to wait until a school vacation. Trust the school staff only if you are *sure*. The trouble with packed lunches is twofold and probably obvious to you at once. The most convenient foods, such as bread, are banned on the diet. Sandwiches are out! Moreover, even if you do send your child off with a tasty and entirely permitted lunch in a box, there is no guarantee that it will be eaten. As every child knows, 'swapping' fare is a perfectly legitimate way of livening up an otherwise boring meal. But that's the last thing you want to happen. Use this approach only if you can trust the child implicitly.

Academic performance

Talking about school meals and teachers makes this a good place to stress again the relationship between food incompatibility and academic performance. I would like to refer you once more to the case of Maxine, quoted in Chapter 10. One of the commonest of all manifestations of allergy reported is a disturbance in concentration and alertness.

Dyslexia may be associated with this phenomenon, and if this were true it would be nice because it would make it very treatable. Certainly when being tested at my clinic, children sometimes react to food and other substances so strongly that they become unable to read and write or to decipher characters correctly: Comprehension is lost, and images may be inverted. One of my young Irish patients called Eamon had an extraordinary reaction to wheat and apple; if he ate either food he would write only in mirror image format – perfectly legible, but in reverse. I tried to explain to his mother the dazzling brain power required for such an extraordinary feat. He was a very bright lad, once this "handicap" was removed.

The trouble with labels like dyslexia, as I said earlier in connection with a 'fancy' diagnosis, is that it detracts from the real cause and implies knowledge of a condition which exists by the mere virtue of giving it a name. There are, moreover, cases where handwriting and word comprehension deteriorate to sheer illiterate nonsense under the effect of a bad allergen. The difficulty comes and goes according to diet, and for this reason the unfortunate child may be judged careless and inattentive at times, or even willfully disobedient, which is most unjust in the circumstances.

Many retarded schoolchildren start to improve enormously in performance as soon as their allergy foods are identified and removed. They were retarded all right, but only by bad diets! It is vital for teachers to be in possession of this knowledge if they are to avoid meting out unnecessary and unwarranted punishment. Obviously, if a pupil were to consume a quantity of food he or she was susceptible to before a class he or she would be likely to be rendered incapable of useful study. This is particularly true after lunch. My estimation of school lunches was never very high, but the modern offerings, with a swing towards fast foods such as sausages or burgers and cans of soda with caffeine and sugar, are a recipe for disaster.

To me there is no more certain way to ruin the potential of a young life than to lay such extreme emphasis on academic performance as we do and yet to expect our kids to succeed while coping with some of the diets that are forced on them. That the education committees concerned serve these foods as a 'convenience' (to them) and an effort to economize is to me intolerable. Are we to sell out the future of our children, their aims and achievements, merely because town hall bureaucrats wish to cut corners in their financial planning?

The trouble is that the majority of public servants who run our lives were themselves no great shakes at school, to judge by their obvious lack of performance in cerebral functions. Perhaps they have 'tame' dieticians who tell them what they want to hear, but by all appearances they scorn advice from concerned nutritionists and listen only to accountants bleating about figures and balance sheets. But of course, even here, the deficient reasoning of the institutional mind is very evident. Cheap, inadequate meals are a complete *false* economy. Rather like 'saving money' by not servicing a road vehicle: in the end, the real cost is many times higher than doing it right in the first place.

The Feingold diet

Hyperactivity in children, also labeled ADD and ADHD, is a new condition *created by* the mass technology of our oh-so-smart society: it was not diagnosed until recent decades. Partly, the reason may have been that no one knew it existed and therefore didn't look for it, but that would only account for a few overlooked cases. The fact is that it is measurably on the increase, and the reason is not hard to find: this unpleasant affliction is a direct offshoot of our deteriorating diets riddled with junk, sugar and chemicals.

There are many degrees of it, of course. Not all cases are severe and debilitating; sometimes the child seems no more than unusually naughty, restless, irritable and unable to sleep a full quota of hours. Parents often fight the diagnosis as if it were something to be ashamed of. Perhaps psychiatrists, who unfortunately usually end up treating the condition, are to blame for not recognizing that it is an environmental disease not a character deformity.

Perhaps it is true also that some of them, hating to admit any of their precious diseases have a merely physical basis, will deny any connection with diet. They would rather treat a child with tranquillizers and soporific drugs such as Ritalin than take the trouble to work out *why* he or she is over-emotional, racing around frantically, hardly sleeping, pale and sickly, with dark rings under the eyes and willful to the point where sometimes it seems he or she is not even under his or her *own* control, never mind that of the fraught, exhausted parents.

Nevertheless, the dietary basis of hyperactivity has been well established by the work of many competent doctors. I myself have seen enough cases recover fully on a simple elimination program to no longer feel the need to question this point. I believe only those practitioners who don't take the trouble to *look* will miss the connection.

One of the interesting and well-known pioneer diets in this field was that of the pediatrician Dr Ben Feingold. He thought he noticed an association between hyperactivity and aspirin-sensitivity in children. If he were right, and aspirin or aspirin-like substances (called salicylates; see page 145) made children hyperactive, then avoidance of these and similar chemicals as food additives should benefit the condition. So he tried putting these children on diets that avoided foods (mostly fruits) which contain natural salicylate substances (these include peaches, plums, raspberries, grapes, oranges, apricots, cucumber and tomato), and was gratified to observe that this produced a measurable improvement. He then went further and suggested the removal of foods containing colorings, preservatives and chemicals. This, too, seemed to be of some help.

The fact that his reasoning was incorrect – at least in my opinion – does not detract from the enormous scientific importance of his contribution to child health. But he made two significant mistakes. To begin with, diets avoiding coloring and so on must of necessity be different in other ways as well: it is a mere assumption to attribute the change to avoidance of chemicals alone. Could it not be due to the absence of *other* factors in junk food, such as sugar, corn syrup or glutamates, which were being omitted at the same time?

Experience suggests it is.

Secondly, Feingold's work did not go far enough. Chemicals *are* a problem to allergic patients - especially to children; but other foods cause much more trouble more often – milk, for instance. Corn is also a serious allergen, and yet it is a widespread ingredient of manufactured food. Why did he not question these too?

So although Feingold pointed the way, his dietary modifications are too limited. Many hyperactive children simply do not improve on the Feingold diet but will do so on the caveman diet, and that is the final condemnation.

Pregnancy

Needless to say, a discussion on children and their allergies ought logically to include a consideration of how the diet applies to pregnant women. There is no reason to avoid the plan because of pregnancy: in fact, quite the opposite is true. It is a depressing fact that these days a great many babies are being *born* with allergies. The mother's eating habits are, unfortunately, often to blame: if she eats badly, and her diet includes many stress foods, the child may be exposed to sufficient quantities to develop reactions to these substances. By eliminating high-risk foods the mother is in effect treating two patients at the same time: herself and the foetus.

As you were told in Chapter 2, studies show that if one parent is an allergy sufferer there is a strong possibility that the child will be one also, and that if both parents are so affected the risk is dramatically increased. Thus if the mother herself has known allergies, and especially if her husband has too, she would be wise to anticipate difficulties for the child and to plan accordingly. This means taking precautions at the outset to minimize the foetus' exposure to allergens.

The way to do that is to follow the *diet wise* plan; it is a low-allergy diet and so makes sense for pregnant women. If it is carried out properly she will not be undernourished, and for many women it actually represents a great improvement in nutrition. Going without bread, pastries and sweets may seem a little harsh at first, but be quite clear: These are *not* healthy foods. They provide no vitamins and minerals but may actually interfere with the absorption of these vital substances. If you eat well from the selection of allowed foods, you will be providing your baby with the best possible nourishment.

Ignore those who say milk is essential in pregnancy. It is not true. Milk is a high-risk food and, as stated in Chapter 6, it is a very unnatural part of our diet. Don't worry about being deficient in calcium: the idea that nature had our species born doomed to lack of calcium, salvaged only in the last few thousand years that we have been tending cattle, is patent nonsense. By all means take a calcium supplement if you wish to be sure – it won't do any harm. But remember, animals don't drink milk after infancy or take calcium tablets, yet their offspring are not born with rubber bones and teeth!

Follow the steps of the program in the normal way. Care is needed only if the withdrawal reactions become quite severe; in that case, ease off by restoring some (not all) of your diet, waiting until things settle down. Then gradually remove the remainder of the banned foods, perhaps one every few days. It takes longer but is less drastic for either you or the foetus. The testing steps are the same, and no special precautions need be observed. However – and this is a *vital* point – just because you are not sensitive to a particular food does not mean that the baby isn't.

Baby reactions

I astonished readers of the first edition of this book (*The Food Allergy Plan*) by telling them that the baby in the womb may respond to food challenge tests!

It is curious and fascinating but not too surprising when you understand the science. Food substances in the mother's blood easily pass the placental barriers and so arrive in the baby's bloodstream. If the foetus is sensitive, it will react in the way most kids do: become hyperactive. Mothers I have coached on this technique were able to tell when the baby was kicking much harder than usual and, by keeping careful records, actually diagnose allergic foods before the baby was born.

Remember the banned foods are likely allergens, so it can he argued that even if you, the mother, don't need to eliminate those foods it would be a good idea to continue doing so for the baby's sake. Investigations show that babies born to mothers on a low-allergy diet have far fewer allergy problems and actually fewer health problems of any sort.

As a final word of interest on this topic, it was one of my patients who suggested the possibility that sometimes when the mother feels ill due to eating a food this might be because of the baby's allergy. It is a fact that sometimes because of her pregnancy a woman begins mysteriously reacting to food that did not trouble her previously. The idea that this could be the reason is new to me, and I haven't yet had the chance to check this out, but the possibility is certainly a most intriguing one.

The first twelve months of life

I carried many babies through their initial diet, from birth to around twelve months old, steering the parents on how to avoid the child developing allergies.

Colostrum, the first sticky mother's milk, is packed with antibodies and very healthy. It seems that if anything other than this colostrum is the first thing to enter the newborn's stomach, then it will be sensitized. So what do they give in hospitals when they snatch the baby from mother's arms? Glucose syrup from corn in a pacifier! Is there any surprise that corn is one of the commonest allergies in children, second only to milk?

Breast-feeding, as everyone knows, is healthier (for the child) and more and more women take this responsibility seriously. Unfortunately, a great many allergens are able to pass through the mother's milk into the child. In this way a baby can sometimes be made allergic to cow's milk and other substances without ever having eaten them. Don't overlook this vital fact, even if your doctor does. An unhappy baby that snuffles, cries a lot, feeds poorly, fails to thrive or has colic (any one of these symptoms or a combination) may be a victim of food allergies *via the mother's milk*. It is a pity that this very helpful piece of knowledge is not more widely known. Untold hours of suffering and frustration on the part of the parents, not to mention that of the baby, could be avoided by a few judicious steps if only someone knew what to do.

This means that if a woman is nursing – and especially if she or her family has a history of allergies or intolerance – she should follow the dictates of this plan. That means, at the very least, avoid dairy produce, corn, sugar, caffeine and alcohol, until weaning is complete.

Once weaned, the child should avoid all dairy produce for a year. Despite all the frenzy for milk and calcium, I have never encountered a child that came to harm by this key exclusion, *providing a good diet of meats, fish, fruit and vegetables was the staple*. On the other hand, I know directly or indirectly of millions of kids who are sickly and suffering because of the inclusion of milk in their diet.

Feedback from patients suggest that I was scoffed at a great deal in the post-natal sessions and by the family physician. But, as before, I was proven right – just twenty years ahead of my time. The American College of Asthma, Allergy, & Immunology developed a consensus document for introducing solid foods into an infant's diet to avoid development of food allergies, and they published the new guidelines in the July 2006 issue of the *Annals of Allergy, Asthma, & Immunology.*

In it they acknowledge that cow's milk and dairy products should be withheld from the diet of infants at-risk of allergy and intolerance. Based on a review of fifty-two studies, they suggested that early introduction of solid foods can increase the risk for food allergy, that avoidance of solids can prevent the development of specific food allergies, that some foods are more allergenic than others, and that some food allergies are more persistent than others. The authors write: "Foods should be introduced one at a time in small amounts. Mixed foods containing various food allergens should not be given unless tolerance to every ingredient has been assessed." [*Ann Allergy Asthma Immunol.* 2006; 97:10-21.]

Incidentally, continuing breast-feeding beyond twelve months seems to carry a slightly *increased* risk of allergic disease.

One step ahead

For those women with time to plan, the best time to look ahead to baby's health is before you become pregnant. It is a curious fact that humans go to a great deal of effort to get animals into peak condition for breeding, and yet we don't trouble to do the same for ourselves. Farmers are very familiar with the fact that sickly, ill-fed stock will breed young in similarly poor condition. Prize animals are given the best of all they require in the way of good food and nutritional supplements before going to stud. I think it is high time we started applying this principle to parents-to-be.

Veterinarians are especially good at nutrition. We could learn a great deal from them.

Obviously, if you are contemplating getting pregnant, *now* is the time to sort out your own personal health and get rid of those harmful foods that don't suit you; the same applies to your partner. After you have conceived may be too late. The reward of a healthy, bouncing child full of energy and free of the sadly common complaints of colic, snuffles, crying attacks, hyperactivity and the whole catalogue of 'normal' childhood problems is surely well worth the effort. You may follow up the dieting regime with nutritional supplements. Just bear in mind that any vitamin or mineral supplement pills and formulas can be allergenic.

For more information on this vital topic of *pre-conceptual* care, contact The Foresight Association. Their address is in appendix E.

Fertility

While we are on the subject, many couples experiencing infertility problems find the answer in diet and nutrition. Food intolerance may be keeping the body functions below par. Sometimes the food intolerance directly interferes with the proper absorption of vitamins and minerals, such as zinc, which are essential to optimum fertility. We call this malabsorption and you can read more about it in Chapter 20.

One of my celebrated cases was a woman who got pregnant after twenty years of trying; she was mainly allergic to milk and her health improved dramatically after I took her off it. The result was a howlingly funny headline in a major UK Sunday newspaper. It said, "I Got Pregnant *After* The Milkman Stopped Calling." It was quite a shock; the lady in question had consented to a press interview in good faith. Her picture duly appeared in the center pages, all smiles, with the new baby. All should have been well, except that some smart young sub-editor got the idea for this headline and it took a lot of arguing from me to convince her I had not connived in a trick. Only copious assurances and flowers saved the day.

Following the elimination diet plan and taking adequate nutritional supplements is probably the best advice to give infertile couples, when no obvious disease factors are present. Remember both would-be parents need to take these steps, not just the woman.

If the risk of having an allergic child is very high and breastfeeding seems impractical or impossible for any reason, soya milk is a *relatively* safe alternative. There are many different brands of this product, and some are better than others. Soya milk, you will realize, is an even less natural substance than cow's milk; therefore it will hardly surprise you to learn that the incidence of allergy to soya is rapidly on the increase as it is used more and more frequently. There is also an on-going debate, whether it interferes with full natural growth.

Believe it or not, it is possible to follow the entire plan given in this book using the elimination and challenge of foods on a breast-fed child via the mother's diet. If she herself follows the diet outlined in Chapter 11 and the fractious, difficult or sickly infant recovers, she can then find out which foods were to blame by reintroducing them one at a time into her eating pattern exactly as if the symptoms were her own. If the return to any given food is accompanied by a deterioration in the baby's condition, that food should be avoided. Foods that cause no problems may be retained in the diet. All the rules given for behavior of food allergies and how to test for them apply when doing this: in other words, it is no use testing the baby by having the mother eat a food which has not yet cleared from her bowel. The five-day period must elapse, otherwise the baby is receiving doses from the mother's colon, via her blood and milk, enough to keep a masked allergy or intolerance in ferment.

If you are a parent, tired and worn out by sleepless nights, give it a try. I wish you luck and the baby many hours of contented rest.

Casebook 11. A child's story

Young Michael, aged eight, was addicted to eating candles and also to eating the black carbon that forms 'round the top of gas stoves. The former he would eat whenever he could get them, which wasn't often since his parents refused to have them in the home any longer. The latter was in plentiful supply, and no amount of vigilance on the part of his mother seemed to be of any avail in thwarting him. Sometimes he would rise in the dead of night, when even the most trusty wardens sleep, and indulge in his unique and disgusting gourmet habit.

If that was strange, it was only a beginning to the sad and complicated tale that his parents unfolded to me. Michael was without doubt mentally subnormal; yet he had not been so since birth. He had made good progress at first and now seemed to be going backwards, though nobody seemed sure why. He was now at a special school. But how bad was his condition? I listened attentively while his father explained that he was deaf; that got me interested. It is almost proverbial to me that deaf people, because they cannot hear and so often fail to understand, *appear* stupid. But when I heard that Michael suffered from recurring unpleasant infections of the ear, nose and throat, that got me *very* interested indeed. Without building up the parents' hopes too much, I suggested that his respiratory troubles might be due to an allergy. The elimination diet could help to locate these allergies, if food were the cause; then his infections might clear up, his hearing *might* improve, and then ... well, we would see.

They agreed to start him on the diet plan. I met these good people several times over the subsequent weeks, and the picture gradually became clearer. Michael, it seemed, was quite a handful. Far from presenting the picture of a low IQ, he was incredibly inventive when it came to mischief: he would turn instructions completely round and do the opposite of what was required. Good with his hands, he had dismantled several objects with a screwdriver, including his own sleeping cot when he was quite young. The fact that he was really subnormal became less and less tenable as a working hypothesis, I thought. He was antisocial and uncommunicative all right, but not stupid.

Well, I'm pleased to say he improved on the diet. His tutors noticed it immediately and were soon asking questions about his treatment. For the first time it was possible to feel that communication was bridging the gap between this lonely little boy and the rest of us. He in turn responded by becoming more playful and affectionate. The exasperating willfulness of his behavior seemed to lessen as he became more contented and better adjusted. His mother told me with some pride that if she now asked for the door to be closed it would be closed, not swung wide. We were winning, though progress was steady and slow.

Food incompatibilities

We eventually established that Michael was intolerant of wheat, milk, sugar and especially colorings and chemicals (tartrazine and others) commonly used in children's pseudo-fruit drinks such as orange squash and 'pop.' Avoiding these substances, which for him were as deadly as poisons, he continued to make good progress.

Subsequently Michael attended one of his regular follow-up visits with the pediatrician managing his case. The gentleman was rightly impressed and most interested in what we had been doing. It was then that he confided to the parents, for the first time, that Michael had been diagnosed as a case of *disintegrative psychosis* (Heller's Syndrome), a wretched and helpless collapse of the child's mind and capabilities being the only considered prognosis. The specialist admitted the mistake, which was generous of him and exciting for us; but I don't think the poor man appreciated the shock this revelation caused the stunned parents.

With such a condemning diagnosis on his records it meant that Michael had been virtually written off. Many encounters with unsympathetic officialdom now seemed to make sense in the light of this new, sinister information. Even a dentist had one day told his mother that there was no need to explain what he was going to do 'because Michael wouldn't understand anyway'. This had astonished her because there had never been any doubt in her mind that her son understood what people were saying!

Luckily this ticket to oblivion was struck from his records, and everyone is very pleased. Michael is now simply ESN (educationally subnormal). He was, inevitably, many years behind in learning, and it would be a fairy-tale ending to imagine that he will one day be normal, and yet...

The children are our future

All compassionate and intelligent human beings love and care about children. They are our future: their bright-eyed innocence, freedom and beauty are the best we have to offer to the troubled world of tomorrow. So, really, their problems are important to us: they affect our own and the human race's survival. Unfortunately, because of our profligate waste and bad husbandry of resources, modern children are in for a tough time of it when they become adults. Our folly has bequeathed them an environment that is full of chemical toxins that pollute the earth, water and even the air we breathe on a scale never before equaled. Already this accumulation of poisons is making many people ill, and unless something is done to halt this Gadarene rush (from the demon-possessed Gadarene swine in Matthew 8:28 that rushed into the sea). I'm sure not any man, woman or child will escape its devastating effects.

For children more than adults, I hope this book succeeds. With so many years before them, sick children need all the help they can get – otherwise they may be condemned to a great deal of unnecessary illness.

Kids grow up!

Remember the obvious: children become adults. In my heyday kids were the emerging problem and my life was filled with looking after them.

But I didn't get to see more than a fraction of the total child cases of ADD and behavioral disorder. Most of them grew up into adults and most of them, of course, still have the problems in later life.

Maybe you suffer from ADD or ADHD? Typical symptoms include:

- a mind which easily wanders off the task in hand
- difficulty concentrating
- impatience and a tendency to try to rush things
- a difficulty bringing order into life's tasks
- scatty thoughts and difficulty remembering appointments etc.

- restless or fidgety
- making hasty decisions which later turn out to be disastrous
- temper outbursts (short fuse)
- mood swings
- always on the go
- a tendency to "drift off" and daydream

If you see yourself in this list, you had better get *Diet Wise*, fast!

Remember ADD does not imply low IQ. Some highly intelligent individuals suffer with ADD.

17

Problem Situations You May Encounter in Elimination Dieting

In this chapter we will consider aspects of elimination dieting, the problems that may arise, and useful solutions to these.

The advice that follows has application both in the initial test phase of the plan and in long-term management of avoidances which may have been found necessary.

Eating out on the diet

One of the most important difficulties everyone encounters right away is the problem of eating away from home. Not many people, even twenty years after I first wrote this book, have much idea of what it means to follow a strict exclusion plan, so you can expect little help or sympathy from restauranteurs or hotel staff.

Part of this is prejudice and part ignorance of the issues involved. Allergies still have the stigma of 'all in the mind,' and even close family might not be sympathetic to what you are trying to do: expect some rebuffs. There is an unfortunate tendency in the population to view a meal such as a chop and vegetables as inadequate eating in some way; it makes many people feel uncomfortable. There is a misconception at large that a 'balanced meal,' supposed to be so desirable, consists of a little bit of everything, including wheat, dairy, sugar and stimulant drinks. So if you are eating with others, expect attitudes that vary from scorn to indifference.

One thing that motivates hostility, I'm sure, is the fact that those you are with also have allergies and addictions: seeing you overcome your cravings will remind them inappropriately of theirs, since they are not able to defeat them. It is rather like giving up smoking: this seems to goad fellow smokers into every level of objectionable behavior. Its basis is envy, plain and simple. If you have ever watched someone try to give up smoking, you may have been struck by the way 'friends' pester, wheedle and even try to trick them into starting again. Clearly, smokers like company and don't want anyone implying their habit is filthy by attempting to give it up.

The same sad rules seem to apply to bad eating habits. Rather than court trouble or hostility from others whose company you keep and perhaps rely on, it is better to be discreet and keep what you are doing to yourself. Just stay at home until you have worked through the program.

Restaurant eating is even more impractical: most menus feature little or nothing without wheat, milk or sugar, and the dieter is left out in the cold. If you can find a place with understanding staff that will cater to your needs, so much the better – enjoy yourself. But the usual reception for anyone who wants to be different is being treated as a crackpot. Quite likely this will offset any pleasure you may derive from successfully eating out. Again, there often arises a need to defend the status quo, as if in saying 'I don't want your food' you are implying it is unwholesome or disgusting. Waiters and chefs are more likely to he hostile than sympathetic, but try it if you must.

One surprise problem in a restaurant environment is that of odors: after unmasking a number of food allergies, it occasionally happens that food odors cause nausea. This is logical if you consider it, but hardly helpful when you are trying to enjoy your meal. Also, general food smells may stimulate urgent cravings for forbidden foods that you find really hard to resist.

On the whole it is better not to dine out during the initial test period, but if you find you must, for business engagements or other reasons, a few simple precautions will prevent you getting into difficulties; after all, the last thing you want in front of a potential client is to be made to look foolish or a crackpot by a smart aleck waiter. First of all, decide ahead of time where you want to eat. Telephone for the menu and find out if there are any *a la carte* items that would suit you. Licensed restaurants are usually able to serve mineral waters or juices. Choose melon (no sugar), avocado (skip the vinaigrette) or smoked salmon (this has usually no coloring) as starters. For the main course you can have fish or meat with salad; just avoid any sauces. It is better to avoid the dessert altogether, or ask for plain fruit.

A helpful *maître d'hôtel* can make your visit as smooth as possible under the circumstances. Just hope you don't hit on an establishment like the one a patient of mine did. A tactful phone call made in advance had appeared to have everything discreetly arranged, but in front of the assembled guests a waiter came up and said in a loud voice, so that everyone could hear, "Ah, You're Mr. So-and-so who phoned up an hour ago to ask for no wheat, milk and corn in your food!"

If you find a good place to eat, stick to it. And if all this sounds rather extreme and oppressive to you, do remember we are talking about a situation you would be better not to put yourself in.

Cafés are hopeless. Snacks in our modern, civilized world seem to consist entirely of tea, coffee, sodas, milk shakes, cakes, pastry, sandwiches, burgers, ice-cream and similar. These are useless to the dieter. If you must travel, stock up with a bag of the things you need and take it with you. Stay away from snack bars. If you are with people who want refreshment in one of these places, have your spring water handy and ask for a glass. If you explain you are on a special diet, not many proprietors would be offended. Some patients are bold: they produce a bag of herb tea and ask for a cup of boiling water. It is easier to pull this off without embarrassment if you are with someone who makes purchases. If necessary, pay the cost of a cup of tea and ask for hot water only.

To a large extent, your own attitude dictates your success in these situations. If you can cope cheerfully through all the vicissitudes and come up smiling, the chances are that things will go your way. If you *have* to make compromises, then do so: that's only being practical, and you shouldn't feel guilty. But don't see that as a reason to abandon the program. Fortunately, most people who have food incompatibilities will improve dramatically even with mistakes in the diet. The chances are that you are such a one, so stick with it. There is, naturally, a world of difference between being forced into a violation through no fault of your own because of circumstances and giving in because of your cravings. The chances are that you will justify the latter to yourself, thinking up perfectly 'valid' reasons why you must do so, but in your heart you will know it is wrong and that you shouldn't be doing it. Again I will stress a comment that appears often in these pages: those foods you find most difficult to give up are the ones most likely to be making you ill. When you know this to be the case, why cheat and perpetuate your suffering?

Vegetarians

Food allergies affect vegetarians like anyone else, perhaps even more so. Does this surprise you? The rule about allergies and intolerance is that the more you eat a food, the more likely you are to develop a reaction to it, so avoiding meat may lead you from one type of unhealthy eating into another. As I said earlier, vegetarians rely heavily on grains and dairy products – which just happen to be the two commonest and most severe bandits foods. So eating them steadily and repeatedly in whole grain bread, quiches, pastas, pizzas, nut cutlets, cheeses – as vegetarians love to do, is just inviting trouble. Even soya is well into the top ten allergens and so tofu and TVP (textured vegetable protein, meat substitute) are also likely to quickly become a problem.

Many who are committed vegetarians for humanitarian reasons eat egg since here the animal does not need to be killed; but once again this is a risky food to those with a tendency towards allergy. Those willing to eat fish have a rather better chance: at least they may ingest plenty of protein without the likelihood of problems, though there are those who cannot tolerate it, as with any food.

Strict vegans have their own difficulties, particularly in respect to animal-based vitamins (B12, for example), but less trouble with allergy *per se*. Grains are the main hazard. Moreover, it is worth pointing out that pulses (peas and beans) contain many toxins, especially if not boiled well, as explained on page 55. It would be wrong to assume they are 'safe' foods without subjecting them to the screening of this plan, especially if you tend to consume a large quantity.

There are two broad approaches I suggest to vegetarians suspected of having food allergies. The first is to follow the diet more or less as given and allow themselves to eat meat, at least during the test period. For most of those who are not inclined to vegetarianism solely on religious or humane grounds this poses an acceptable temporary measure. There is an advantage in this approach, namely that eating foods not normally eaten, even if commonplace to the rest of us, is rather like switching to exotic foods. The chance of an allergic reaction to allowed foods becomes even further reduced: certainly, if one did occur, it would be noticed at once. This approach enables the patient to avoid more of the regularly eaten foods without starving.

The second alternative is to use a fast or half-fast approach. It is drastic but will give correct answers if carried out and interpreted correctly. The half-fast would consist of one vegetable and one fruit, instead of meat; otherwise, all the information given in Chapter 14 on fasting applies in full. If you really can't face even a half-fast, follow the elimination diet with allowed food that you feel like eating. But it is very important to maintain variety: don't eat several foods over and over again, or you may make yourself ill due to *those* foods.

My experience with vegetarians is that they tend to be keen on diet alternatives anyway and adapt to new ideas rather easily. The reason vegetarians can quote statistics showing they are, in the main, healthier than the rest of us has to do, I think, with the fact they are conscientious and careful about what they eat (rather than the fact that meat harms one). Most of them gave up eating junk food long ago.

The main point of resistance, if I can call it that, is that some vegetarians find it hard to believe that their cherished whole foods can indeed be making them ill. But remember, I commented earlier that it is rather difficult to get *true* whole foods these days. Whole wheat may be whole, but is it also soaked in chemical sprays added to the crop before harvesting and sometimes also in storage. If you react to wheat this might be the reason, so it will pay you to test foods correctly by my method.

Take a day off from your food exclusions!

Here's a useful tip. You can give yourself an occasional rest from food exclusions. A drug called sodium cromoglycate (Cromolyn or Nalcrom) was developed to prevent certain types of allergic response (MAST cell breakdown). Unfortunately, it really doesn't work if you keep taking it. But if you use it just now and again, it will provide enough protection to allow you to indulge your food desires, once or twice a month.

Take it for the day leading up to the anniversary treat or whatever "food holiday" you are planning. Take it the next day, to provide continuing cover. Then stop. Give it a rest for a few weeks.

Dose: take one 200 mgm capsule four times aday, before meals. Open the cromolyn capsule(s) and pour all of the powder into one-half glass (4 ounces) of hot water. Stir the solution until the powder is completely dissolved and the solution is clear. Then add an equal amount (one-half glass) of cold water to the solution while stirring.

Drink all of the liquid to get the full dose of medicine.

Do not mix this medicine with fruit juice, milk, or food because they may keep the medicine from working properly.

Caution: this is a prescription only medicine and your physician will tell you to be careful if you have a history of kidney disease or liver disease.

Alcoholic drinks

It is not widely appreciated that alcoholism is principally a food allergy problem, a surprising insight I gained from the late, great Theron G. Randolph. What the addict really craves is his or her allergy food, not alcohol; it is simply that the alcohol gives the dose more kick. The real 'fix' is with the ingredients, such as corn, wheat, sugar and yeast. Malt of course is sprouted and fermented barley (but may sometimes refer to wheat or rye).

All alcoholic drinks contain brewer's yeast. Wine otherwise contains only grapes. This is the reason you rarely hear of alcoholics who drink only wine: the alcohol content of beer may be lower, but there is nothing in wine that gives the same grains and sugar "lift" as lager, stout, pils and beers. Spirits give a bigger effect still, and many alcoholics soon progress to whisky, vodka and gin. I demonstrated this to my own satisfaction nearly thirty years ago and have found nothing to change my mind.

I did this by giving alcoholics shots of pure ethyl alcohol: it didn't satisfy their cravings, whereas doses of the appropriately administered foodstuffs, such as wheat or corn, immediately relieved the withdrawal symptoms.

Something else I learned, following from Randolph's original teaching: people react differently to different alcoholic beverages. A person may be ill on whisky, fine on gin, suicidal on rum and so on. It is very important to identify a safe tipple, if possible.

Casebook 12.

A man I met in Spain, middle-aged and very portly, was exceptionally fond of vodka. Let's call him Abe (he was Jewish). Abe had had several heart attacks and considered himself lucky to be alive; every day he woke and thanked God with a prayer at sunrise. But a very short conversation with him (at his own bar!) revealed he was almost certainly intolerant of wheat and that this was the cause of most of his health problems, including the obesity. I pointed out that most modern spirits are made from wheat or corn (or both) and that even vodka was no longer normally made from potato. Drinking spirits when you have a wheat allergy is a *bad idea*, I explained to him.

Well, Abe was a connoisseur of vodka and had over fifty brands on his shelves, including many very expensive authentic Russian vodkas. So we went through all the bottles, then and there, and I had him remove the ones that were not pure potato. That left fewer than a dozen.

"Drink those," I told him.

Well, no one could say Abe was weak-minded; his health problems had stemmed from ignorance on his part (and that of his regular doctor), not self-indulgence. He subsequently followed my advice exactly (only visitors got the grain vodkas) and within months he had shed over fifty pounds and felt great. His physician also reported objective signs of improvement. I lost touch with Abe, soon after leaving Spain and returning to live in the UK.

Alcoholism

Actually, it isn't the alcohol that causes the physical ill health of addicts, either. Cirrhosis of the liver and pneumonia are probably the two main causes of demise associated with alcoholism when it reaches dire proportions. The reason the liver is damaged is that it lacks certain essential nutrient ingredients, namely methionine and choline. These are normally supplied in the diet, but alcoholics are notorious for not eating and – despite a frequent appearance to the contrary – it is malnutrition that is their undoing, *not* the alcohol per se. This so lowers their resistance to debility and disease that pneumonia claims a victim where these days it normally would not.

If you are an alcoholic – that is, if you can admit it to yourself and want to do something about it – use the elimination diet plan.

But you should also take large doses of vitamin B3 (niacin): 2,000 to 3,000 mg. a day. These levels are not dangerous but may cause an unpleasant flush as a side-effect, rather like sunburn. Take also a good multivitamin formula; vitamin B1 particularly gets depleted by alcohol and lack of it causes depression and demotivation.

Eat often: do not allow yourself to become hungry. Have a substantial breakfast consisting of fried food, such as liver, chops, kidneys and fish, with one or two extras like mushroom or tomato. Thereafter, eat something every couple of hours. It need not be a great quantity, but you must guard against low blood sugar (see Chapter 19). If you should trigger off this condition, it will bring on an irresistible craving for an alcoholic beverage. At the same time (though it is not as important as the 'drying-out' stage), take multivitamins. This overrides instructions not to take vitamins during the plan; take lots.

Guard against stress and *fatigue* as far as possible during drying out. Your worst danger times are late afternoon and evening when you become tired.

Once you have overcome the period of withdrawal and cravings, it will be easier. Many symptoms from the self-inventory list will probably have disappeared. This should encourage you. However – and this is important – I do not recommend that you try food tests for at least a month. Try instead to continue on the elimination step for that length of time, eat well and stay well. The risk in testing foods is that you inadvertently trip a craving reaction and you are driven back to the bottle. So soon off it, you may find this too much to handle. It is better to improve your general condition with safe eating, rest and vitamins for *as long as you can stand it*. Some people have been on the Stone Age diet for years, so it isn't impossible – it only seems that way at first!

Alcoholics attending my office were surprised (and delighted) I did not make coming off a condition of treatment. In fact the opposite: I tried to ensure the patient was ready for the big step first. I would get him to eat well and take plenty of nutrients, to repair some of the damage. Then, using office test procedures, I established the main allergens and then banned those one by one.

If you want to do something similar, you could arrange a cytotoxic food allergy test, which can be done by sending away blood. The method is not 100% accurate, by any means, but is better than no information at all.

The Internet is a rich resource for finding laboratories that supply this service (ignore the laughable and bigoted website called Quack Watch that comes up on Google).

Diabetics

Many cases of diabetes turn out to be due to food allergies. It is even possible in some cases to conquer the disease so fully that insulin injections may be dispensed with. The dietary type, managed with hypoglycemic drugs such as glibenclamide (Diabeta®, Glynase® and Micronase®), should certainly respond well. Nevertheless, it is important to take care when approaching this condition with alterations in diet. If you suddenly remove a lot of carbohydrate food from your eating (which, in effect, the elimination diet does) you could find yourself in difficulties: in other words, suffering from hypoglycemia attacks in which you could fall unconscious. This is especially true of patients taking insulin, unless the dose is reduced in accordance with the drop in carbohydrate intake.

It is vital to let your doctor know what you are doing in advance. He or she should be able to reduce your insulin dose. If you are the type of patient who is already managing his or her own insulin levels, that makes things much easier. Even so, the condition can become very unstable for a while, and frequent visits to the family practitioner are suggested. As always, you may meet with scorn and attempts to talk you out of any self-diagnosis plan such as this diet. Don't be put off: you may even teach your doctor something!

Steroid medicines

One of the most dangerous groups of drugs in the modern doctor's arsenal are arguably those classified as corticosteroids, not just because of what they may do to the patient but more because of what they take away. They suppress the body's immune reactions and may eventually undermine this important defensive mechanism so completely that the individual is left with little or no resistance to fight even the most trivial of diseases.

Unfortunately, these are commonly prescribed in combating allergic responses.

Nature has endowed us with a superb combative screening system which constantly does battle on our behalf with toxins and microbes that enter via skin wounds, the mouth, lungs and other parts of the body. The white blood cells are part of this system, and their wonderful power to render harmless and ingest all manner of potential pathogens is well known to anyone who has studied elementary physiology at school. Antibodies, too, play a part by inactivating foreign matter called antigens. These are of great concern to us in the study of allergies since some allergy reactions at least are precipitated when antigens and antibodies meet. It is as if the furious tussle with the intruder upsets the furniture and makes a mess, which we call a *symptom*.

That is where steroid drugs come in. With certain illnesses, such as allergy reactions, arthritis, colitis and asthma, the battle is almost too much for the body and needs quieting down. Indeed, with rheumatoid arthritis and other 'collagen' diseases, the whole war seems rather pointless since, so far as we can tell, the body is attacking its own protein! Until the 1950's we were helpless to intervene in these situations. Then therapeutic successes began to be observed with a (then) 'miracle drug' called ACTH. This is actually a hormone that stimulates the adrenal glands to produce their own hormones, which are basically corticosteroids. Our adrenal glands are remarkable organs lying just above the kidneys. They are endocrine, that is to say ductless, glands and secret hormones directly into the blood. The inner layer or medulla produces adrenalin. The outer layer or cortex produces a number of steroid hormones – hence the name corticosteroids. Modern drugs are usually synthetic copies of these substances, derived by chemists from the basic formula.

Steroid hormones have a number of complex actions, which are far from fully understood, including effects on sex and vitality, glucose metabolism (see Chapter 19), the distribution of fat and the density of bones. Yet their most startling property is the suppression of immune reactions. An acute inflammatory focus such as an arthritic joint settles down quite dramatically when one of these hormones is administered; similarly, asthma attacks dissipate, eczema fades and colitis becomes manageable – all this to the obvious relief of the doctor and patient.

Bad trade off

The trouble is that all this success has an important tradeoff: you cannot suppress one type of reaction without doing the same to all the rest. Thus the ability to fight bacteria, which is an important and necessary sort of inflammation required to keep the body healthy, is concomitantly diminished. Furthermore, the adaptability of the body's systems to cope with toxic foreign substances is compromised; thus food and chemical intolerances get worse. Far from being a wonder drug, as they appeared at first sight, steroid hormones are actually a deadly two-edged blade that may often do more harm than good; certainly as a long-term cure they have little to offer.

One of the biggest problems with steroids is the 'rebound effect' which occurs when they are discontinued. It is a very unfortunate fact that even if a disease is firmly controlled by such a medication, when the drug is stopped the complaint flares up again, sometimes worse than ever. In other words, there is a 'Dead if you do; dead if you don't' sting in the tail. Doctors, I'm afraid, fall into the trap all too easily in their enthusiasm to be able to offer some sort of help, and it is true that, for many conditions, steroid drugs offer an attractive, if dangerous option.

Recognition

You may be unaware of the fact that you are taking a steroid-type medication. If you think this may be the case, ask your doctor and get him or her to explain. (Drug) names to look for are words including 'cort' such as Ledercort, hydrocortisone or Efcortelan. But many are much more obscure, such as Depomedrone.

A number of well-known creams and ointments are basically steroid preparations, such as Betnovate, Dermovate and Synalar. Look for the generic names betamethazone or dexamethazone. Incidentally, do not be assured that active drugs are not absorbed from the skin when used as unguents; they are, and this is of special concern with babies, who may absorb enough in relation to their tiny body weight to constitute a *serious* overdose. Many doctors do not seem to realize this important point. Probably the best known of all steroid drugs is prednisolone. The most widely prescribed is the birth control pill, which often is not thought of as a steroid at all.

The advice you were given in connection with the drug may also give you a clue. It is important not to cease taking the drug suddenly. Often recommendations are given to reduce the dose steadily by one or two tablets a day. If when doing this symptoms recur, you can be fairly certain you are taking a steroid preparation.

If any glucocorticoids are given orally or by injection over a period of more than a few days, side-effects common to this class of drugs may occur. These can include:

- Stomach upset, increased sensitivity to stomach acid to the point of ulceration of esophagus, stomach, and duodenum

- Increased appetite leading to significant weight gain

- A latent diabetes mellitus often becomes manifest. Glucose intolerance is worsened in patients with preexisting diabetes.

- Immunsuppressant action, particularly if given together with other immunosuppressants such as ciclosporine. Bacterial, viral, and fungal disease may progress more easily and can become life-threatening. Fever as a warning symptom is often suppressed.

- Psychiatric disturbances, including personality changes, irritability, euphoria, mania

- Osteoporosis under long term treatment, pathologic fractures (e.g., hip)

- Muscle atrophy, negative protein balance (catabolism)

- Elevated liver enzymes, fatty liver degeneration (usually reversible)

- Cushingoid (syndrome resembling hyperactive adrenal cortex with increase in adiposity, hypertension, bone demineralization, etc.)

- Depression of the adrenal gland is usually seen, if more than 1.5 mg daily are given for more than three weeks to a month.

- Hypertension, fluid and sodium retention, edema, worsening of heart insufficiency (due to mineral corticoid activity)

- Dependence with withdrawal syndrome is frequently seen.

- Increased intraocular pressure, certain types of glaucoma, cataract (serious clouding of eye lenses)

- Dermatologic: Acne, allergic dermatitis, dry scaly skin, ecchymoses and petechiae, erythema, impaired wound-healing, increased sweating, rash, striae, suppression of reactions to skin tests, thin fragile skin, thinning scalp hair, urticaria.

- Allergic reactions (though infrequently): Anaphylactoid reaction, anaphylaxis, angioedema (highly unlikely, since dexamethasone is given to prevent anaphylactoid reactions).

Other side-effects have been noted. Ask your doctor, if you notice them and if they are more than mild.

[Source: http://en.wikipedia.org/wiki/Dexamethasone]

How to proceed

With all this bad news, if you are taking a corticosteroid, you will want to see if you can reduce or stop this as a result of tackling your allergy problem. Extreme caution is required, but that is not to say you should not make an attempt, or several attempts, to do so. In hitting at the root cause of your illness it is perfectly logical to expect to be able to manage without any further treatment. It is important to tell your doctor what you propose to do. Only the very poorest practitioner, barely clinging onto the status of a healer, would oppose you in your wishes. A good doctor can be a great support through what may be a difficult and certainly trying time.

The essence of coming off steroids is to steadily reduce the dose. There are bound to be repercussions, and it is hopeless to expect to succeed without at least some flare-up of symptoms. Thus you should wait until the plan shows some sign of working for you before you start. On the other hand, don't wait too long, because the administration of steroid drugs will cloud the issue when it comes to testing and self-diagnosing your allergies.

Be patient: you may have to try many times. There will be failures in which you are forced to return to a higher dose because of unpleasant consequences, but each time you should be able to come nearer to your objective. If there are any criteria which you can measure, so much the better; this may help by giving you a yardstick of progress. For example, an asthma patient may be able to chart the number of uses of nebulizing inhaler; as the need declines, this would show on the daily record.

Similarly, a colitis sufferer might measure bowel evacuations. It is surprising how, on occasion, things progress without a patient feeling any different; the objective measures will help him or her to know whether to continue in a given direction or retreat.

SUMMARY

a. Eating out on the diet is difficult and likely to compromise the stringency of the elimination; it is better to avoid doing so. Take food with you when you travel; plan ahead at a restaurant.

b. Vegetarians are affected by allergies in much the same way that the rest of us are: likely foods relate to frequency of eating. The elimination stage is more restricted because of the unavailability of meat and fish for dietary use. The principles apply in exactly the same way.

c. Alcoholism is basically a problem of *food allergies,* which is alcoholics' true addiction. Good nutrition is important. The avoidance of hypoglycemia (see Chapter 19), fatigue and stress is vital to conquering this condition. Unfortunately, most have wrecked lives and suffer from too much stress to ever escape the addiction. It is all but impossible to help an alcoholic who isn't motivated to help him or herself.

d. Diabetes responds very well to the *diet wise* approach. The elimination diet is very low on carbohydrates, and adjustments may need to be made in insulin levels in order to avoid hypoglycemic faints.

e. *Steroids:* If you are taking this type of drug, coming off it needs care. There will probably be a reactive flare-up, no matter how well you are doing on the plan. Take it by easy stages: wait until each flare-up settles down before progressing to the next increment down in dose. Vitamin and mineral supplements are vital at all stages.

18

Let's Talk About Substitutes!

Now, having spent so much time in the previous chapters dwelling on what not to eat, it's time we turned to the positive and looked at what you can eat.

There is no question that when deprived of corn flakes, bread, tea, coffee, muffins, pasta, pizza and so forth that people start to panic slightly.

"But what *can* I eat?" was the question I probably encountered most. Usually it was said in such woeful tones that the interrogator clearly believed there was no reasonable and redeeming answer likely to be forthcoming.

So we will celebrate the kitchen in this chapter. I will offer you a variety of suggestions for what to eat, to show you what can be done. You can use these as a starting point and learn to make your own way, following your own preferences in what to eat and how you like it prepared.

These are necessary skills I'm afraid because, as I taught the majority of my patients, "I may cure you of migraine (arthritis, colitis, urticaria or whatever) but I can't cure you of allergies. It's a tendency you will always have and you need to live with it." Nowadays this is even more true, when we take genetic food intolerances into account. You can suppress the faulty genes by eating properly, as I have suggested. But those genes are still there and will manifest once again if you start to take too many liberties.

Substitutes

The key to it all, of course, is substitutes. If you can't eat a certain food, what could take its place? In the early eighties, it was a much bleaker situation than today. With the rise of health food stores and supermarkets enriching the possibilities by importing exotic foods from all over the world on a constant daily basis, things are much easier today. This is equally true in the USA.

When we lived in south Manchester in the remains of a large manorial estate, I ran my office from home. My young pre-teen son, both entrepreneurial and a skilled young cook, spotted a market immediately and offered to serve my patients a variety of tasty cooked lunches, which would conform with the dietary restrictions – wheat-free, milk-free, corn-free etc. He made a few dollars and learned what was to be a very valuable trade. He grew up to be a prize winning chef, with his own magazine column, working in Michelin-starred restaurants.

The point of saying that is to be able to say that most patients were delighted and surprised at what could be done, without the common and seemingly "indispensable" ingredients found in the average kitchen. He came up with a great many soups, salads, pot roasts and even a few desserts, to show that the case is not a hopeless one, and that if a young kid can do it, most people can.

Ingenuity and creativity are required but not unrealistic culinary skills that would be beyond the abilities of a typical adult.

Consider flours (farina): today it is possible to get flours made from buckwheat (not wheat and not in the grains family), potato flour, gram flour (garbanzo), sago flour, tapioca flour, chestnut flour and many others. Wheat is highly prized, for its gluten content, which makes it sticky, especially suited to bread and cake making. Rye, oats, barley and triticale are also gluten foods and available as flours but they contain much less gliadin, which is the fraction of gluten that makes wheat sticky.

The trick is to learn to cook differently. Fluffy loaves may be out but scones and pastry can be made to work, with some care.

Dairy substitutes

There was a time when the only substitute for cow's milk was from the goat or sheep. Goat's milk has acquired an almost mystic reputation over the centuries for curing diseases, from eczema, to colic, asthma to catarrh. Sickly children were often switched to cow's milk in the old days and usually made a full recovery. I can now tell you why, with certainty: *goat's milk creates a cow's milk exclusion!* Goat's milk does little or nothing positive. But it does keep a body off cow's milk and that's where the recovery comes from. Just remember you read it here first!

The truth is, about half the people who react to cow's milk also react to goat's milk. Almost certainly, in this instance the allergy is to the casein protein and ewe's milk will also be a problem.

On the other hand, some individuals are allergic to the phospholipids fraction; the fatty part. They may possibly tolerate skimmed milk, which has most of the fat removed.

Instead of walking a tightrope, it may be better to follow a completely dairy-free path. In this case, look for milk-like substitutes from differing sources.

Allergy and intolerance isn't the only health problem with milk. For a more comprehensive report on other health hazards in milk, take a look at a stimulating website called www.notmilk.com. I agree with most of what you will read there.

Lactose intolerance

Still others, as you may have heard, are not exactly "allergic" to milk but have a lactose intolerance. That means they lack the enzyme called lactase (*alactasia*), which the body uses to digest lactose in the gut. Typical symptoms of this deficiency are abdominal pain and discomfort, bloating and wind. The difficulty comes when new-born babies suffer lactose intolerance. They may experience profuse diarrhea which can lead to life-threatening dehydration and loss of vital electrolytes (body chemicals). Early research into this problem was carried out in Manchester (UK) by my old professor Aaron Holzel and we now understand the condition a lot better. Special formulas are available for these infants and usually treatment is begun even before they are discharged from the obstetric unit. Incidentally, I dated Holzel's daughter Helen – just for one evening!

Lactose (milk sugar) accounts for a startling twenty-five per cent of all carbohydrate in the average Western diet. It is present as forty per cent of milk solids (cow's, goat's and ewe's). This percentage rises to over fifty per cent in skimmed milk and whey but is less in whole cream and yoghurt. Butter and cheese have almost no lactose.

Commercial buttermilk is usually made by fermenting skimmed milk, which effectively reduces the lactose level of the skimmed milk by some ten to fifteen per cent. However, buttermilk may have added dried or condensed milk, which would of course alter the proportion of lactose.

Lactose intolerance test

Where the onset is less serious and the symptoms less dramatic, *alactasia* may go undiagnosed for years.

The simplest proof of lactose intolerance is a lactose challenge test. The patient fasts, then consumes 25 mg of lactose, the equivalent amount to around 0.5 liter (about two cups) of milk. No other foods or drink are allowed for the subsequent three hours, during which time the patient is monitored for the development of symptoms of intolerance, such as gas, abdominal cramps, bloating, or diarrhea.

The results are not always reliable and several repeat testings may be wise before the diagnosis is dismissed outright.

More sophisticated testing may include a biopsy of the intestinal mucosa and an analysis of its lactase activity.

Treatment

For the majority of people, avoiding lactose is the best course of treatment. Most adults, with a little attention to detail, can get all the nutrients they need without recourse to milk, though since the problem is less serious than an allergy this exclusion need not be comprehensive.

If you feel you *must* have dairy products, they may be predigested or taken with a lactase supplement, such as Lactade®.

Hidden lactose

It isn't always easy to recognize lactose in manufactured foods. Whey is obvious, but sometimes even this is disguised as 'emulsifiers.' Lactose may also be present in 'milk-free' infant formulas, in sweets and fudges; even in bread.

Conversely, hard cheeses and cream may be well tolerated, as may be plain (dark) chocolate. However, cottage and cream cheeses do contain significant amounts of lactose, since they are not fermented.

Prolonged boiling reduces the lactose content of milk. However, pasteurization is too short a process: these days just fifteen seconds (minimum) at 162 °F/72°C.

Sweeteners

Patients often ask what can be used for safely sweetening foodstuffs. My preferred answer is *nothing:* just change your palate. Even a carrot tastes very sweet, once you have given up sugar.

However that may be too extreme and I myself do not follow a strict exclusion. Sweet treats can be delightful, now and again. But not too often.

The important thing, I think, is to be properly informed.

Firstly, understand there are many forms of "sugar." High fructose corn syrup (HFCS) is notorious and a widely used additive to food. You will likely encounter it in manufactured foods more often than actual sugar. What's the problem? you may ask. Fructose comes from fruit, so it's nice and healthy and natural, right?

The answer is a resounding NO.

A team of investigators at the USDA, led by Dr. Meira Field, has discovered that fructose is not so human-friendly. The researchers wanted to compare the health effects of fructose and glucose, so they fed two separate populations of study rats on either glucose or fructose. The glucose group was unaffected but the fructose group had disastrous results. The male rats did not reach adulthood. They had anemia, delayed testicular development, high cholesterol and heart hypertrophy. The key to this, the researchers believe is that fructose in combination with copper deficiency in the growing animal interferes with collagen production. Copper deficiency, incidentally, is widespread in Western society. The females were less affected, but they were unable to produce live young. [Fields, M, *Proceedings of the Society of Experimental Biology and Medicine,* 1984, 175:530-537.]

All this is very reminiscent of Frances Pottenger's experiments on cats I have already drawn to your attention (page 53). Pottenger's Cats, as they are known, soon became sterile on the wrong foods.

If that were not enough, the rats also developed cirrhosis. "The medical profession thinks fructose is better for diabetics than sugar," says Dr. Field, "but every cell in the body can metabolize glucose. However, all fructose must be metabolized in the liver. The livers of the rats on the high fructose diet looked like the livers of alcoholics, plugged with fat and cirrhotic."

Moreover, because it is metabolized by the liver, fructose does not cause the pancreas to release insulin the way it normally does. Fructose is metabolized only very slowly and so converts to fat more easily than any other form of sugar. This may be one of the main reasons Americans continue to get fatter.

It also seems to be liver toxic, at least in the form it's served by manufacturers. So you would not want to eat HFCS in any drinks (sodas), in any food, *ever*.

Real sugar

Let us then return to the subject of real sugar.

Familiar cane sugar (white or brown) is in the grass family (grains) and therefore a relative of wheat and corn. Beet sugar is available but, whereas once you could be sure which was which by purchasing a specific label, that is no longer true. Tate and Lyle once supplied cane sugar exclusively; now they will buy whatever is cheap in the market on the day. The same is true of other suppliers.

Beware of labeling tricks. Aware that people know raw brown sugar has at least *some* nutritional benefits (a few minerals, is all), manufacturers now make artificial "brown" sugar. It is white sucrose colored with dyes. Avoid "soft brown sugar" or any similar labels; just look for authentic names like Demarara or Muscovado, a British specialty brown sugar, which is very dark brown and has a particularly strong molasses flavor.

A good tip I used give patients is to look for the "country of origin"; if it says Guyana, Brazil, or some such, the chances are it is real raw sugar. If it says "manufactured in Celveland, Ohio" or something similar, the chances are that it isn't.

Honey

A lot of people get dewy-eyed about honey. It comes from reading *Winnie the Pooh*, I expect, rather than looking at science papers.

Let me state clearly: *honey has no real health advantages over natural sugar sources*. It is sweet, sticky (rots your teeth) and contains about 80% sugar, as follows:

- Fructose: 38%
- Glucose: 31%
- Sucrose: 1%
- Other sugars: 9% (maltose, melezitose)

In view of the remarks I made above about fructose, it is hardly a desirable product, except as a very occasional treat. The same is true for natural honeycomb. But it does taste very good, I must admit.

Manuka honey is another story altogether. It seems to have powerful anti-microbial qualities. But don't let tht blind you to the fact it has a very high glycemic index.

Bee pollen, "Royal Jelly" and propolis are very different, even though they have a related taste and come from the same source.

Watch out for added sugar in commercial cheat brands. That rather defeats the purpose.

Stevia and the rest

A number of plant sweeteners, such as Stevia, from a South American shrub, have come onto the market and enjoy a certain popularity. I'm sure there will be others in time. Though Stevia can impart a sweet taste to foods, it cannot be sold as a sweetener because the FDA considers it an unapproved food additive. The subject of searches and seizures, trade complaints and embargoes on importation, Stevia has been handled at times by the FDA as if it were an illegal drug. Under provisions of 1994 legislation, however, Stevia can be sold as a "dietary supplement," though it cannot be promoted as a sweetener.

Whereas one might suppose these herbal sources are "natural" and therefore healthy, I have a problem:

Stevia is some 300 times sweeter than sugar; Talin, a protein found in berries grown in West Africa, is 2,000-3,000 times sweeter. That's seems very unnatural to me! All these foods do is create a palate raving for extra sweetness. Use them if you must. But surely, I have always taught patients, it is better to accustom your palate to *less* sweetness. After a time, the natural sweetness inherent in foods will emerge and you'll find you don't need sugar-substitutes nearly as much.

Sugar alcohols

Though not technically considered artificial sweeteners, sugar alcohols are slightly lower in calories than sugar and do not promote tooth decay or cause a sudden increase in blood glucose. They include sorbitol, xylitol, lactitol, mannitol, and maltitol and are used mainly to sweeten sugar-free candies, cookies, and chewing gums.

FDA classifies some of these sweeteners as "generally recognized as safe" and others as approved food additives.

Finally, the filth

I'm reluctant to even mention the items in this section in a book on human health and probably risk being heavily sued anyway. But I do feel it is right for me to issue the warnings; it's up to you whether you heed them or not.

On no account should you allow aspartame sweetener in your diet or that of anyone you love or care about. None.

There is abundant scientific evidence to link aspartame and glutamates to serious degenerative diseases, such as Alzheimer's, Lou Gehrig disease and Parkinsonism. Yet this substance is added as a sweetener to countless sodas and food. Whenever you see the label "lite" or "diet" soda, that would usually mean aspartame.

Did you know aspartame works fine as a poison for ants? Just spread the powder on the floor, wait till they retrieve it and see them vanish. With fire ants apparently you have to add a little moisture to dampen it, before they will take it back to the nest. Within two days all evidence they ever existed is gone.

It's beyond belief that this substance was ever passed as safe for human consumption. In fact the FDA opposed it for years – until President Reagan had his man installed as the FDA Commissioner, who promptly passed it as safe, despite all the studies which showed differently.

The same can be said of a product called Splenda™, the brand name for sugar-derivative sucralose, made by UK sugar giants Tate and Lyle. They cutely say it is made from sugar and is therefore "natural." Nothing could be further from the truth. Splenda™ is converted from cane sugar to a chlorinated no-calorie sweetener which isn't recognized as sugar by the body and therefore is not metabolized. Anyone with an understanding of basic biology would know that is a very dangerous thing to put in your body. Just because it is of no use in healthy metabolism does not mean it cannot get into our body chemistry and mess things up. In fact sucralose *raises* blood levels of the main diabetes marker glycosylated hemoglobin (Hba1C); that's the one thing you want to keep *down* in diabetics.

Moreover animal studies show that sucralose fed to animals can lead to damage to the liver and kidneys, spleen, thymus and lymph glands, reduce growth and provoke problems with pregnancy.

The claim that sucralose passed adequate safety tests is disingenuous at best, criminal more like. Only six trials were ever carried out on humans and only two of the trials were completed and published before the FDA rushed to approve sucralose for human consumption. In those two trials only thirty-six human subjects participated and only twenty-three were given sucralose. *The trials lasted only a matter of days and only looked at sucralose in relation to tooth decay, not human safety and tolerance!*

Kwok's Queaze

A favorite medical Finals examination question in my day concerned what was sometimes called the "Chinese restaurant syndrome" or "Kwok's Queaze," presumably after a Chinaman named Kwok, though whether he was made ill by it or the doctor who first wrote about it, I cannot say.

It was an unpleasant reaction to monosodium glutamate, including headache, nausea and flushing of the skin.

Kwok's queaze was considered a specialty item then, a tricky question to pick out the possible honors students; today I notice that there is barely a reference to the queaze which shows up on all of Google, presumably because MSG-induced symptoms are so familiar.

Egg substitutes

Eggs, as stiffeners and binders, are pretty essential in cooking, so if you can't eat egg without reacting to it, then you need a substitute.

An egg is made up of various proteins, several of which are highly allergenic. One of them, ovalbumin, is the major allergen and makes up fifty percent of an egg white so you *may* be OK with egg yolk.

Commercial egg replacers are available, such as *Ener-G Egg Replacer* (suitable for vegetarians). Just follow directions on box. Make sure you identify the listed ingredients; Bipro, for instance, is whey protein isolate and would not suit anyone intolerant of milk and derivatives.

But you can try many natural foods as egg replacements. I have seen nice waffles made without egg, without milk and without flour (well, no wheat flour); they were made with gram flour and soya milk! Gram flour (from the garbanzo bean) binds very nicely.

Yoghurt, mashed banana, applesauce, pumpkin, or other pureed fruit or vegetables are good replacements for eggs in muffins or cakes.

Use the following table as a guide:

2 tbsp arrowroot flour = 1 egg

2 tbsp potato starch = 1 egg

1 heaping tbsp soy powder + 2 tbsp water = 1 egg

1 banana, mashed = 1 egg in cakes or muffins

Bread replacements

Last but not least, what can you do when bread (wheat) is an issue?

Long known as the staff of life, bread is actually a food that causes a great deal of ill health due to the widespread prevalence of wheat allergy and intolerance. There is also a great deal of misleading propaganda from manufacturers. An example is their use of the term 'improvers' as an ingredient. These additives fluff up the loaf to make it lighter; that means you are sold more air and less bread.

Another deception is the redefinition of 'wholemeal.' Traditionally this sort of bread contained only wholemeal flour, yeast and something to texture the rough grain (usually soya oil or similar). Due to an increasing interest in healthy eating in the 1970s, more and more people began to turn to this kind of loaf and abandoned commercial white bread. What did the manufacturers do? They lobbied to have a law passed relaxing the legal definition of wholemeal so that they could sell an inferior product to the unsuspecting public under the label 'wholemeal.' Now, since 1984, bread only has to *contain* wholemeal flour to be called wholemeal.

I shock many people with a paradox, which is contrary to the accepted propaganda: white bread may be safer for you than whole grain! Many wheat-intolerant individuals cannot eat the whole grain product but the refined loaf has less of the characteristics of 'wheatness' and so may not provoke any allergic response. If you are one of these individuals, try to get a simply made white loaf from a small local baker. They tend to use fewer ingredients and bake a better product anyway.

Avoid loaves guaranteed 'fresh for days.' The ideal loaf for allergics is one that is uneatable the next day and has to be bought daily, as the French do. A loaf that is too poisonous for mold and bacteria isn't very healthy for humans, after all.

Wheat-free breads

Those intolerant to wheat in all degrees will have to try wheat-free bread. Unfortunately, even most rye loaves also contain wheat. Rye on its own is very leaden and unappealing, but the exception is German moist black rye bread or "pumpernickel," which is usually wheat-free. In any case, I'm told you cannot crop rye without getting at least some wheat seeds included and the resulting stems and ears will "contaminate" the rye.

Years ago there was little else to offer but nowadays it is possible, with a little sleuthing, to track down breads made from sago flour, tapioca, rice and other flours. Always remember the texture is not so good because of the lack of gluten, the magic cooking ingredient!

Some of these loaves, it must also be said, are exceedingly expensive for what they are. Usually I try to encourage patients to just do without bread, rather than maintain a longing at great expense.

Don't forget simple rice cakes will stand as a good pinch hit for bread. These are rather boring (like polystyrene ceiling tiles is the usual joke) but will take butter and jam, or cheese or a slice of ham as well as a slice of dear old bread.

You can always try rye crackers (Swedish crispbread).

Yeast and mold allergy

A common incompatible food is yeast. This is often accompanied by mold sensitivity and there may also be a *Candida albicans* infection, which is a whole issue in itself.

Yeast-sensitive patients need to avoid yeast and mold contacts. A complete list is given in appendix B.

We consume a lot of molds inadvertently – not just in cheese and mushrooms – unwanted molds. Bread is a shocking and surprising avenue of exposure. In 1980 the following fungi were found in flour milled in the UK: *Penicillium, Cladosporium, Aspergillus candidus, Aspergillus flavus, Mucor, Aspergillus terreus, Alternaria, Aspergillus versicolor Absida, Aspergillus fumigatus, Verticullium* and *Paecilomyces* (Food Surveillance Paper, HMSO, no 4, 1980).

Mold contamination of animal feeds can lead to further exposure. Both molds and toxins (along with antibiotics, hormones and sedatives) pass into dairy produce, meat, eggs, bacon and poultry.

As the molds' main port of entry is the mouth, the digestive tract tends to be the most affected. Darkness and moisture within the gut suit these organisms very well. Add to that the fact that our immune systems seem to be already under siege and, not surprisingly, we have a formula for trouble of epidemic proportions. Malabsorption syndrome develops due to intestinal inflammation together with an inability to eliminate cellular waste. As my friend Dr. Nancy Dunne in Dublin was inclined to put it, 'Pseudo-celiac disease with negative alpha-gliadin antibody titres and normal jejunal biopsy but full symptomatology is now as rife as the common cold"'!

If you cannot eat yeast but wheat is safe your problem is different. You'll need to make soda bread. The commercial kind usually contains buttermilk, which is fermented and not allowed on a yeast-free program. Actually, after a bit of practice you will be able turn out a very palatable product.

Making soda bread

This traditional Irish soda bread is surprisingly quick and easy to prepare. For one 8-inch loaf you will need:

1	tsp butter/dairy – free margarine/oil
1	lb/455 g flour
1	tsp bicarbonate of soda/baking soda

1 tsp salt

4-8 oz/115-225g buttermilk/goat's milk/soya milk (water if you are stuck)

Preheat the oven to *hot* (475°F/220°C). Grease a large baking tray and set it aside. Sift the flour, soda and salt into a large mixing bowl. Gradually beat in the buttermilk or other liquid. The dough should be smooth but firm. If necessary add more and shape it into a flat round loaf, approximately one and a half inches thick and eight inches in diameter. Place on the baking tray and with a sharp knife make a deep cross on the top of the loaf. Place the loaf in the oven and bake for 30 to 35 minutes or until the top is golden brown. Remove from the oven and allow to cool. Best served slightly warm.

19

Testing For Allergies

Some of you may be tempted to skip the "trial and error" approach and go for laboratory testing. That's bound to be quick, easy and accurate, right?

Unfortunately, no. There are no good blood tests that reach even 50% validity.

Even the food challenge test—eating the food to see what happens—is not a good test method, unless carried out exactly as I describe it here. There are often false negatives (a bad food is missed). So the idea that a food challenge test should be the real benchmark of food reactions doesn't entirely hold true.

But when we come to laboratory tests, the results are even more unreliable. Let me lay it out for you.

The two main test routes are:
- conventional allergists and their immunological approach
- alternative lab testing methods.

Conventional testing may be appropriate for you, if you have one of the very narrow range of allergies which can be detected this way: mainly these are Type I hypersensitivities (for skin scratch and antibody tests) or Type III and IV hypersensitivities (for patch testing). For reasons of completeness, an overview of these methods is included here. But the essential drawback of this route is that, at the end of the day, no matter what is found, you are going to get the same basic treatments: drugs and medicines. The conventional allergist has little else to offer you and, as they pompously pronounce in their own position papers, do not sympathize with the kind of self-help philosophy expounded in this book.

If you are seeking something more than just pharmacology, you may feel that taking this old-fashioned route is rather a waste of time. It's up to you. You could of course try a combination approach and the next few sections might help you understand better what is being offered.

Conventional Allergy Testing Methods

Prick or scratch tests and hyposensitization

The mainstay of conventional allergy test has not advanced significantly since 1911, when the prick and scratch test method was first developed. For this method a small drop of the substance being tested is dropped onto the skin, which is then scratched or pricked with a needle at that spot. The amount of flare and wheal compared to that caused by a control (inert) solution gives an indication of how allergenic the substance is (Noon L., Prophylactic Innoculation against Hay Fever, Lancet 1, London, 1911, p. 1572).

It is a very inaccurate method, with many false negatives, and subjects seldom react to food at all in this way, though a demonstrable allergy may be present on challenge testing.

An important migraine study at the Great Ormond Street Hospital for Sick Children in 1983 showed that none of the cases would have recovered by following an exclusion diet based on the results of the prick testing included in the trial, though 93 per cent improved on a suitable diet, showing that food allergy was the cause (Egger J. et al. Is Migraine Food Allergy? Lancet, London, 15 Oct 1983, pp.865-8).

- False negatives: are disastrous because you are misled into believing the substance is safe
- False positives: are merely inconvenient, you avoid something unnecessarily, when it is quite safe

One final failure, which is not talked about: the substance with the largest reaction may not be the one which is causing you the most trouble, as I have found out many times with the help of Miller's Method (see later in this chapter, page 225).

The hyposensitization method aims to find out which substances the patient is allergic to, by giving a whole batch of prick testing, and then to administer injections of a mixture of these, increasing gradually in strength, until quite large amounts are being tolerated. The body is often then found to be able to cope with normal ambient concentrations.

There are two major drawbacks to this hypo-sensitization treatment:

1. it rarely works and
2. it can be extremely dangerous. Patients sometimes react severely and deaths due to anaphylaxis occurred regularly until by common consent its use was abandoned in 1986, except in special circumstances and where full cardio-pulmonary resuscitation equipment is at hand.

The only suitable indications for the use of this method are in cases of perennial rhinitis and asthma due to dust and dust mite allergy, seasonal rhinitis due to pollens and the danger of anaphylaxis due to insect stings. Even so, very brittle (vulnerable) cases, especially children, are better left un-desensitized, since the dangers of the method are very real.

Immunological tests

Other conventional allergy tests are based on immunological reactions of the IgE antibody type, or occasionally IgA and IgG. Naturally, classic antigen-antibody reactions are the only results to be expected, which precludes a large number of other allergic and intolerant reactions.

Broadly speaking, then these tests are fine if they give a positive result; which is to say, if an allergy to wheat or egg is found, it probably exists. Avoiding that food will help with the overall body load. But negatives are meaningless (these occur over 95 per cent of the time when foods are being tested). Also, a positive reaction on an immunological test only means antibodies are present, it does not mean the allergy is the one causing symptoms. Experts often overlook this elementary point.

The RAST (Radio-Allergo Sorbent) Test

This is the basic immunological test using labeled molecules for quantifying results.

Specific antigen (in this case the allergy being tested) is incubated in contact with a plastic plate or tube until it becomes bound by adsorption (adhesion).

The plate is washed and the patient's serum, with suspected IgE antibody to that allergy, is added. This naturally locks on to the antigen. Unused sample fluid is washed away, leaving "captured" IgE.

How much IgE antibody has been captured is measured by adding a second binding antigen, in this case radio-active anti-IgE, which locks onto the IgE in the antigen-antibody complex. This creates an antigen-IgE-antigen "sandwich".

After unused labeled molecules have been washed away, the amount that remains behind can be measured using a gamma counter (Geiger counter). Hence: radio-allergo sorbent test or RAST.

Another variation called the ELISA test (enzyme-labelled immuno sorbent assay) is to label the anti-IgE with a color-generating chemical (enzyme). After washing, adding a second enzyme releases the dye. Sensitive spectrometry measures how much color is now present, hence giving an indication of how much IgE is present.

This approach gives an exquisitely sensitive measurement of how much antibody was present in the serum being tested, using only tiny amounts of test solutions.

Trouble is, there are so many false negatives, particularly with food reactions. This is partly what has fueled the myth that food allergy reactions are rare. IgE is only one aspect of the allergy and intolerance phenomenon and only a small part at that.

Conclusion: orthodox allergy testing for foods is virtually a waste of time and resources. Even if you get a positive, the treatment offered is not holistically-based but pharmacological.

Non-Conventional Allergy Testing Methods

These can generally be classified as the good, the bad and the downright awful. Remember that the value in the test method may lie as much in the treatment which goes with it as the actual technique itself. For that reason I introduce first an entirely scientifically credible testing option, which gives good accuracy and leads to a treatment method that has spelled freedom and health for countless patients.

I myself have taken over 10,000 people through it over the decades since I was shown it. This is how I made my amazing discoveries, like the Irish boy allergic to potato (page 83). Conventional allergists fight it tooth and nail, entirely through vested interest. The controversy rages on. You are provided with some references to clinical trials in the appendix, which you may pursue for yourself.

Other "alternative" methods you may encounter are described in here outline. You can find more details on my website at: www.alternative-doctor.com

Miller's Method (provocation-neutralization)

Also known as serial end-point skin titration, this is the method that enabled me to find some remarkable and obscure allergies, which would otherwise probably have remained hidden.

It was first developed by Carleton Lee of Missouri in the late 1950s. Lee began a series of investigations by injecting his allergy patients with antigens at different concentrations. He noticed something interesting: sometimes he provoked a symptom, which wasn't surprising, but sometimes a patient's symptoms would disappear over the space of just a few minutes, which was very surprising indeed. It was one of those lucky situations where the right person is in place, at the right time, to draw useful scientific conclusions. Lee realized immediately that diluting an antigen could make it effective at neutralizing the symptom associated with the allergy.

In fact it emerged that only one specific dilution had this serendipitous effect, which Lee christened the "neutralizing dose"; unfortunately, it is different for each patient (and each allergen) and has to be tested individually. But it is a major advance and offered much symptomatic relief for suffering patients. Herbert Rinkel and others went on to improve Lee's method and promote its more widespread use, and the first definitive book explaining the technique in detail was written by Joseph B. Miller (Food Allergy: Provocative Testing and Injection Therapy, Charles C. Thomas, Springfield, Illinois, 1972); hence known as Miller's method.

Lee's widow has (quite rightly) campaigned to have it recognized as the Lee-Miller method.

The Method

After testing the control and being assured of the zero baseline reaction, a food test reagent (or dust or chemical) is injected superficially into the skin, making a deliberate wheal. If this grows compared to the control over, say, 10 minutes, this suggests an allergy. The bigger the wheal, the more probable the culprit up to a point. Thus far it looks like scratch or prick testing; but because of the safety factor implicit in the explanation below, we use quite concentrated reagents, which cause foods to show up often, unlike with the scratch or prick method.

Sometimes a symptom is produced (provocation) and this is much more conclusive. Remember these substances are tested one at a time, so there is usually no doubt which food caused the symptom.

If a reaction occurs (wheal or symptom), the patient is then given a series of weaker and weaker injections of the same substance at 10-minute intervals until the wheal ceases to grow and the symptom, if there is one, disappears completely.

This 'switch-off' dilution, the first non-growing wheal, is called the neutralizing dose; it works as a kind of antidote. The procedure is illustrated in the figure.

1st dose wheal 1	2st dose wheal 2	3st dose wheal 3	4st dose wheal 4
◯	◯	◯	◯
8x8	8x8	8x9	8x10

wheal 5	wheal 6	wheal 7	neutralizing dose wheal 8
◯	◯	◯	◯
12x13	10x10	8x9	8x8
Symptoms patient experiences discomfort	**Symptoms** worse	**Symptoms** lessened	**Symptoms** gone
Wheal hard raised blanched	**Wheal** hard raised pink	**Wheal** soft raised pink	**Wheal** soft level pink

The size of the wheal at start is unimportant

Safety note: Even very unpleasant symptoms are brought rapidly under control by injecting a more dilute dose of the allergen (nearer the end-point). Final adjustment of the correct end-point means that symptoms have vanished altogether. In over half a million test doses I only ever once encountered anaphylaxis, which was blocked by immediate administration of epinephrine (adrenalin). At the time of writing no death has occurred due to Miller's method, despite its use by thousands of doctors world wide. This is in sharp contrast to the hypo-sensitization method, which caused multiple deaths annually until discontinued.

Nevertheless it is sensible to avoid injecting any substance into a patient who has already had an anaphylactic reaction.

Sublingual Neutralization "Drops"

After testing a number of substances, a patient can then be given a cocktail of the resulting neutralizing doses. These are administered as sublingual "drops"; one drop under the tongue, shortly before food will usually allow the patient to eat the food safely. This is in contrast to strict avoidance, if no kind of desensitization is attempted.

Obviously common sense must play a part and if the reaction is severe, reduced intake may be necessary. But it is better than a life of strict avoidance. Happy patients have found themselves able to eat and drink troublesome items and so rejoin social life on virtually equal terms with the rest of us.

When we first started using this approach in the late early 80s, it was of course scoffed at. I was called fraud by more than one doctor. But it is satisfying to report that the medical profession has caught up at last and sub-lingual immunization therapy, or SLIT, is now widely practiced. You can find thousands of pages devoted to it on Google, if you enter this search term.

Problems

When it works, the method works very well. A number of difficulties may occur, however. About 10 per cent of cases are plagued with shifting end-points. Repeat testing becomes necessary and this is troublesome and may be expensive. These shifts can occur very rapidly. So that by the time the patient is supplied with his or her prescription, it is ineffective. In these cases, even retesting won't help. However, this only applies to less than 5 per cent of those tested.

Unfortunately, the people who need this kind of treatment most, the very sick, 'unstable' patients, are the ones most likely to be troubled by this shifting end-point phenomenon.

Even if the antidotes are not effective, however, the method is still good for diagnosis. It can pinpoint rapidly the worst allergens for a patient. This will help reduce his or her body load. The method is also very safe.

Reactions are common but rarely severe, and in any event can be relieved rapidly by the corresponding neutralizing dose.

Sublingual Provocation

A modification of the Lee-Miller technique is to do the testing sublingually. This dispenses with syringes and the need for a physician altogether. A food or other concentrate is placed under the tongue and the reactions noted. If the patient experiences a symptom, this is neutralized, as before, by serial dilutions. The dilution that switches off the symptom completely is taken as the end-point (Dickey, LD Sublingual Use of Allergenic Extracts (monograph) ed. H C King, Elsevier, New York, 1981).

There is no essential difference between this approach and using an injection, although naturally there are fewer parameters by which to judge reactions or the lack of them. Instead of being able to view a wheal, its size and characteristic, the clinician has only the patient's subjective symptoms to rely upon, plus what he or she can observe objectively.

Yet with practice it is possible to become quite adept at spotting subtle shifts in the patient's mood or attitude, skin colour, etc. The neutralizing dose would be that which leads the patient to declare his or her symptoms 'switched off' and the clinician to note that whatever manifestations arose have disappeared again.

Controversy

No technique of clinical ecology has been more heavily criticized than Miller's method. Nevertheless, most of us who use it do so because we are aware of its capabilities and accept its scientific validity. More and more papers are being published that show its effectiveness. Yet the controversy won't go away.

Over the years a number of studies have been cited to show that Miller's method is a fake. Almost without exception these have been improperly reported, evidence for key statements has been missing and data has been altered (or withheld) or the protocol so bad that it was obviously designed to invite failure.

In 1973 the Food Allergy Committee of the American College of Allergists, using sublingual provocation testing (see below), carried out a study that showed that the neutralization basis of Miller's method was quite effective. Did they publish their findings? No, they repeated the whole test again in 1974 and this time found that the statistics were not as good. The second study was therefore termed 'The Final Report' while the first positive study was simply cast aside.

The 'Jewett trial' carried our in 1981-83 was appallingly defective. The results remained unpublished for seven years, so clinical ecologists world-wide were deeply shocked when it was suddenly published in August 1990 in the New England Journal of Medicine. This, the world's second most prestigious medical journal, even went to the extraordinary length of issuing a press release announcing that at last the clinical ecologists were going to be sunk. I won't say such spite is without precedent in medicine, but it certainly has no place in a scientific periodical.

To my mind, Miller's method is an outstanding contribution to medicine. Like all medical techniques, it requires skill if it is to be performed correctly.

Cytotoxic Tests

This next method sounds closer to the classic antibody blood tests, such as the ELISA test. However there are significant differences and it is far from mainstream yet.

Use of a white blood cell toxicity test for food allergy antibodies was first recorded by P. Black in 1956. The test at that time was crude and produced results that are best described as suggestive, rather than conclusive.

Since then, methods have slowly improved. The technique is simple but depends for accuracy upon a high standard of laboratory technique and even then could not be said to be accurate.

White blood cells are separated by centrifuging, placed on a microscope slide chamber and mixed with about 10 mg of food extract. The sample is then observed at intervals over the next two hours and the effect of the food extract on the white cells is noted.

Healthy white cells are mobile and exhibit amoeba-like behavior. On contact with an allergen however the cells lose their mobility and become rounded in shape. Cytoplasmic granules become sluggish and cease to stream. Eventually, damaged cells rupture and die. Hence the name for this procedure which is cyto (cell)… toxic (damaging).

Results are typically reported as red foods (do not eat); orange foods (eat only occasionally); and green foods (safe to eat).

Scaling

It is customary to grade reactions from 0 to 4, depending on severity of damage, observing the following changes:

0   reduction or loss of amoeboid movement
1   intracellular stasis (slow-down or stop-page)
2   rounding and distortion of cell contour
3   vacuolation (the appearance of tiny vacuoles, or cavities)
4   cell lysis (bursting open)

Dr. Damien Downing, who first introduced this method into the UK, claims that it has an 80 per cent accuracy. There are many critics however, even among clinical ecologists, who do not take these claims seriously and who point to many well-conducted trials which show that the method is virtually useless. Cytotoxic testing appeared to suffer a mortal blow to its credibility when, for a stunt, journalists sent blood from the same person on the same day and received two widely different reports on the fake patient's sensitivities.

The real difficulty with the test, in common with many other methods, is that it rests in the final analysis on human interpretation rather than objective measurement. This isn't so bad as long as each laboratory is at least consistent with its own standards. But it may, on occasion, lead to patchy quality in results, which can be very misleading for the patient.

Modern test systems, such as the ALCAT or Nutron test claim to get round this element of observer error by using mechanized counting. My experience is that there are still far too many false negatives.

The LEAP Test

The latest incarnation of cytotoxic testing is the LEAP test (lifestyle eating and performance). It is said to be more accurate because is measures volume changes in the white cells, rather than a 2-ddimensional microscope image.

Probably the main drawback of the cytotoxic test method is that it needs intelligent and knowledgeable back-up by a competent doctor. Otherwise the patient is left avoiding certain foods indefinitely, with no clear place in mind, struggling to keep up an adequate diet n a selection of things to eat that may be pitifully limited.

Unfortunately, this after-care is not always readily obtainable and the laboratories themselves often duck the issue.

Applied Kinesiology and Related Methods

This method of testing for allergies usually raises a few medical eyebrows. AK testing is a kind of body dowsing.

It has its origins partly in chiropractic and partly in acupuncture and was first described and developed by George Goodheart in the USA. As its name suggests it is primarily concerned with the dynamics of posture and movement . Although it has no proven scientific basis it does seen to be founded on a certain body wisdom. A simpler version for the layman, called Touch for Health, was developed by California practitioner John F. Thie.

Allergy testing is only a small aspect of this discipline. Applied kinesiology is based on the discovery that if the body is subjected to adverse influences, certain muscles go weak. No-one pretends to know the physiological basis of this effect, simply that it can be shown to exist.

The kinesiology practitioner gauges the strength of a group of muscles (techniques exist to improve the tone of weak muscles and generally balance the body's dynamic status before starting). Then, by putting a sample of food under the patient's tongue and retesting, he or she is able to tell whether body is adapted to that food. In fact it isn't necessary for the patient to take in the food; just holding some will work just as well.

If the muscles weaken significantly, the food is deemed to be an allergen.

My main criticism, having dealt with innumerable patients who have been first to a kinesiologist and had a failed or only partial result, is that the majority of AK practitioners are naïve in being unaware that their own body reacts too. So many of these people diagnose "wheat allergy" or some other reaction on virtually everyone who enters their office. Like all "dowsing" techniques, it is a case of find what you want to find, unless you take vigorous steps to try and prevent this auto-diagnosis.

The Auriculo-Cardiac-Reflex Method (ACR)

Even stranger technique than applied kinesiology, but one I have learned and seen perform well, is the auriculo-cardiac-reflex method, developed by French neurosurgeon Paul Nogier.

It is based on the fact that stimulation of the sympathetic nervous system causes the rate of maximum pulse amplitude to shift along the artery. Note: this has nothing to do with pulse rate, which does not necessarily alter.

The test is calibrated as follows: the practitioner rests his or her thumb over the radial artery at the wrist so that the impulse is just out of reach beyond the tip of his or her thumb. A bright light is then shone onto a sympathetically enervated portion of skin, either the earlobe or the back of the hand. This causes the point of maximum amplitude of the pulse to move till it comes directly under the practitioner's thumb.

Done properly, it is like feeling nothing until the light shines, at which point the pulse suddenly starts to bump under the counting thumb. This response to light is called a positive reflex. Once established with a patient, then it is sought as a sign of an allergen (actually, just a sign of sympathetic stimulus, which is not quite the same thing).

Testing foods and other allergens is simply a matter of holding a filter containing each substance over the skin of the forearm. A positive auriculo-cardiac reflex lasting a dozen or more pulse-beats is a sign of an allergy. If it lasts 20 or more beats, that is a severe allergy.

With set of filters covering common foods and other allergens, it is possible to test quickly a wide range of substances. Once again, the patient must simply avoid the food but, since only the most pronounced allergens show up, it doesn't usually lead to a long list of banned substances.

As with the applied kinesiology method, the ACR technique is a fast and cost-effective means of allergy testing, sacrificing high accuracy for expediency but a very useful method, nonetheless, particularly with children.

Postal Allergy Testing

Sometimes you will see advertisements for "allergy testing", where you send a blood spot, spit or a hair sample. You need to be aware that these tests are pendulum dowsing (or similar). I have no problem that dowsing can work, in the right hands. At $20- $50 it's not exactly robbery, even if done badly! But I think it only right that dowsers make it clear that is what they are doing and not leave it vague, so that worried patient believe it's more scientific than it is.

20

Malabsorption and Leaky Gut

Remember your intestinal tract is just another organ. It has a pretty complex task, which is to break down all kinds of foodstuffs and turn these into metabolizable fuel for the cells. Think of it a bit like the way ancient pine forests were decayed and turned into fossil fuels, such as oil and coal, but much much quicker – in a few hours instead of millions of years.

It does this by means of chemical reagents we call enzymes. These are remarkable substances which enable complex chemical processes to take place quickly at body temperature; where normally such transformation processes would take a very long time or require a source of heat, such as a Bunsen burner – the normal chemical reaction you would see in a test tube at High School.

In the mouth, ptyalin (salivary amylase) is added to our food, a starch digester, which begins to break down carbohydrates, even as we chew. Also in saliva are lysozyme, an enzyme which attacks bacteria, and IgA antibodies, a class characteristic of the whole intestinal tract.

In the stomach hydrochloric acid is secreted, together with pepsin, which starts to break down proteins and rennin, for the digestion of milk. One other important stomach secretion to mention is *intrinsic factor*, without which we cannot properly absorb vitamin B12. Lack of stomach acid (called *achlorhydria*) often goes along with B12 deficiencies, which leads to a condition called pernicious anemia (because it really was fatal, until all the causes were discovered). I can tell you that achlorhydria (no acid) or hypochlorhydria (not enough) are quite common in patients with food allergy and intolerance and may lead to a similar B12 deficiency.

As soon as the sloppy food mass reaches the next section of gut, the duodenum, then two more very important organs come into play: the pancreas and gallbladder. The pancreas adds some industrial-strength enzymes, for the digestion of fats, proteins and carbohydrates. At the same time secretions turn the liquefied food back to an alkaline mix, or chyle, as it is known. The gallbladder is really a liver storage reservoir and bile salts are secreted by the liver, not by the gallbladder. Bile acids are vital because they enable fats to emulsify. This term means fats in suspensions as tiny droplets in the watery liquid (milk is an emulsion).

The duodenum (which literally means "twelve fingers," from its dimensions) has been likened to a second stomach. It is a good analogy. Many animals, as you know, have more than one stomach. Most of the digestive process takes place here, leaving mainly simple sugars, amino acids, simplified peptides and fatty acids. From there on down the rest of the gut, absorption is the name of the game.

The wall of the small intestine is lined with tiny hair-like growths, which increase the absorption area. These can be damaged, causing difficulty in absorption. If the loss of functional capacity is severe enough, as in celiac disease, the patient may simply waste away and die. Nowadays we know the cause is gluten allergy and by avoiding gluten, the individuals' gut returns to normal and absorbs quite satisfactorily.

Finally, the large bowel (colon) absorbs most of the fluid content, compacting food into feces, ready for expulsion. The familiar color and smell come from the breakdown of bile acids into two compounds, indole and skatol and the putrefactive process, releasing hydrogen sulfide, methyl mercaptan and ammonia.

Nobody (to my knowledge) treats the smell of feces; it's not as critical diagnostically as smelly urine. But if you should wish to reduce the odor of your feces, be advised that proanthocyanadins from grapeseed extract will do just that, and do it very well, according so a study published in 2001 [Jun Yamakoshi, Shoichi Tokutake, Mamoru Kikuchi, Yoshiro Kubota, Hiroyasu Konishi, Tomotari Mitsuoka, Effect of Proanthocyanidin-Rich Extract from Grape Seeds on Human Fecal Flora and Fecal Odor, *Microbial Ecology in Health and Disease*, Volume 13, Number 1/February 1, 2001].

Green tea also has measurable but smaller effect in reducing offensive odors in the stool.

See also the box on Flatulence, page 000)

Three main problems

If you want to know more about the digestive process and the functional anatomy of the alimentary canal, I suggest you check out one of the many available texts. I merely introduced this outline sketch of what takes place in the gut in order that you may understand the rest of this chapter, which focuses on three principal ways in which things can go wrong:

- The digestive breakdown process may malfunction, leading to incomplete digestion. This results in foodstuffs being absorbed in a form capable of setting up specific allergic or intolerance reactions.

- Malabsorption, which means that proper nutrients are not taken up from the bowel, as they should be, or not in sufficient quantities, leading to impaired nutrition.

- Lastly, the gut may absorb digestive refuse that it would be better not to do, a problem we call "leaky gut."

These evils do not occur on a one-or-the-other basis, but tend to come together in varying degrees. Indeed food toxins and allergens can *cause* malabsorption and leaky gut, because of their destructive effect on the intestinal living. Let us take each in turn and see how it relates to food reactions and overload.

Enzyme deficiency

Many people with food intolerance have impaired digestion. Incomplete digestion of foods which then pass through a leaky gut into the bloodstream is a major contributing factor to the problem of food allergies and genetic food incompatibility. It means recognizable food molecules are spread throughout the body and are thus very likely to set up adverse reactions. The resulting antigen-antibody complexes may settle in any organ and cause symptoms related to that organ, a process similar to what we call "serum sickness," which was seen after incompatible blood transfusions and still turns up occasionally after injection of drugs or antidote sera.

There are several things you can do to improve your digestion. The most basic is to pay attention to how you eat. Take your time; chew your food very thoroughly. Apart from the fact that ptyalin enzyme is added in the saliva, chewing breaks the food down into smaller particles that can be acted on more easily during its passage through your digestive system.

There is a prevalent belief that swallowing liquid along with food "dilutes" the enzymes needed for digestion. In reality, studies have shown that a moderate intake of one to two glasses of water with a meal improves digestion by facilitating both the production of gastric secretions at the time you eat and also the secretion of bicarbonate into the small intestine that normally occurs one to two hours after a meal. [Bland, Jeffrey, Ph.D. *Digestive Enzymes*, Keats Publishing, Inc., New Canaan, CT, 1993, p. 9.]

Understanding the role of the digestive tract leads to a hypothetical way of improving food tolerance which is to ensure more complete digestion. We can do this by adding supplementary digestive enzymes. This would be strongly suggested if you can identify food particles in your stools.

Digestive enzymes are available as supplements in several forms. Pancreatin is an extract of the pancreas of cows or pigs and is a very potent, broad-spectrum aid for the digestion of proteins, fats and carbohydrates. However, if you are allergic to beef or pork, you will probably not tolerate pancreatin.

Broad-spectrum plant enzymes are derived from the fungus *Aspergillus orazeae*. They are also active in the digestion of fats, proteins, and carbohydrates. Milder but very useful plant digestive enzymes are papain (from papaya) and bromelain (from pineapple); the two are usually combined in a single preparation. The latter only really digest proteins, not fats and starches. Just remember that you can become sensitized to plant and animal enzyme sources, just as you might a food.

To avoid this problem, Dr. William Philpott, one of the leading developers of this technique, recommends the rotation of digestive enzymes on a four-day cycle, using pancreatin (from pork and beef), plant enzymes from *Aspergillus orazeae*, bromelain and papain in turn. [Philpott, William H., M.D. *Victory Over Diabetes*, Keats Publishing, Inc., New Canaan, CT, 1983, p. 69.]

I have outlined several suggestions for digestive enhancement later in this chapter.

Hydrochloric acid

Along with digestive enzyme lack, deficient hydrochloric acid secretions in the stomach, complete (*achlorhydria*) or partial (hypochlorhydria), is a common accompaniment. This condition also leads to digestive impairment. Its main cause is antibody production against parietal cells, the cells that normally produce the acid, and is therefore an autoimmune disorder. Chronic alcoholism is also a recognized cause. Finally, as we age, we secrete less and less stomach acid until, by the age of 60, around 30% of the population has achlorhydria. An extra complication is that the stomach is no longer rendered sterile but bacteria can flourish, causing further damage to the stomach and duodenal lining. Lack of stomach *intrinsic factor*, which aids absorption of vitamin B12, can lead to pernicious anemia. Finally, if that is not enough, cancer of the stomach is more prevalent in individuals with hypochlorhydria.

Stomach digestion takes place at a pH as low as 2.0. This is an acid strength capable of burning the skin and damaging fabrics. The arrival of acidic stomach contents in the duodenum is a trigger for the secretion of pancreatic enzymes and bile. These secretions are very alkaline: pH 8.0 or more, because of the presence of large quantities of bicarbonate. pH is a logarithmic scale (4.0 is ten times more acid than 5.0; 3.0 is ten times more acid than 4.0) and so readings of these magnitudes mean that digestive fluids are millions of times stronger than ordinary body fluids, which hover very close to 7.4 (otherwise you die). Just remember these details next time someone tries to persuade you that acid vs. alkaline foods influences body chemistry!

The Heidelberg Gastrogram

This simple test has revolutionized the diagnosis of hypochlorhydria. A holistic physician should be able to arrange this for you.

The patient swallows a small capsule, which is in fact a pH detector and radio-telemetry device. To trigger the acid response the patient is asked to swallow water and sodium bicarbonate. The capsule then measures the stomach pH changes over time and then broadcasts it back to the receiver. The resulting recording we call a gastrogram. The capsule passes through the body and is excreted.

A simpler, cheaper but far less accurate alternative test consists of swallowing a similar capsule or impregnated pad on a string, which changes color at different pH readings. The capsule or pad is retrieved by simply hauling it back up the gullet.

Surprisingly, a common symptom of hypochlorhydria is heartburn, or "acid indigestion." Television commercials tell us that when we have heartburn we should neutralize our stomach acid with various antacids, or, even more drastically, take medications such as ranitidine, cimetidine, nizatidine, or famotidine, which reduce our production of stomach acid. For those who have heartburn because of hypochlorhydria, these medications may lead to further deterioration of digestion and thus to dysbiosis, leaky gut, food allergies and even stomach cancer. You would be wise to work with your health care provider to make sure that the diagnosis is correct: either too much or too little stomach acid.

Digestive supplements

Now that we have looked at the digestive process in a little more detail and seen the effect of inadequate digestion, the reader will ask what can be done.

First try bitter herbs. These stimulate the secretion of stomach acid and digestive enzymes. Angostura bitters are present in many cocktails and the French swear by their aperitif before eating. Examples of medicinal bitter herbs include: Dandelion, Yarrow, Mugwort and Chamomile, which are mild, and Wormwood (as in Absinthe), Barberry, Gentian, Rue and Tansy, which are pretty grim.

You must use a liquid tincture, otherwise the bitterness effect does not trigger secretions. Add up to 3 ml of the herb tincture to room temperature or warm water and sip. Drink 15 to 30 minutes before eating. Another option is to buy an herbal tea containing bitter herbs and drink one cup before eating.

If bitter herbs are insufficient, next try betaine hydrochloride capsules with pepsin. These should be taken at the start of a meal, and the dose depends on the size of the meal. Capsules are preferred. If you take tablets, avoid all contact with the teeth, as hydrochloric acid will damage the enamel. Put the tablets on a spoon and drop them in the back of your mouth before swallowing.

Betaine hydrochloride should not be taken by people taking cortisone, NSAIDS or aspirin, or individuals who have a known peptic ulcer. If abdominal pain, burning, discomfort or dark stools occur, it should be discontinued immediately.

A fuller enzyme regime

For those with complex food intolerance, clear evidence of malabsorption and recognizable food particles in the stool, I suggest you try a fuller regime, based on the recommendation of allergy pioneer Dr. William H. Philpott.

To succeed with this you will need to monitor the state of the acid-alkali process that is taking place in your body. Actually this can be quite simply done by testing the saliva. Suitable pH testing strips are available from familyhealhtnews@amazon.com

Supplement as follows:

Thirty minutes before your main meal take two tablets of pancreatic enzyme extract.

At the commencement of the meal test your saliva. If the pH is higher than 6.0 (inadequate hydrochloric acid), take betaine hydrochloride or similar acidic replacement. Start with one capsule or tablet and increase by one each day.

At this time swallow the pepsin supplement, if you are using one. It is far simpler to have your HCl and pepsin combined in a single supplement.

After the meal: take two more tablets of pancreatic enzyme extract.

Thirty minutes after the end of the meal: take a further tablet of pancreatic extract, a tablet of bromelain with papain, and a half teaspoon of alkali salts mix (sodium and potassium bicarbonate).

At bedtime: take five tablets of pancreatic enzyme extract and two bromelain with papain tablets.

If you have a mind to do so, Philpott recommends a further dose at 2 a.m.: take five tablets of pancreatic enzyme extract, two tablets of bromelain with papain.

I consider this redundant and stressful. Sleep is more valuable than popping supplements.

It's important to use such an enzyme supplement program short term. If you tackle your diet problems properly, as I have outlined consistently throughout this book, you should not need to take enzyme supplements for more than a few months to a year. Take a regimen of vitamin C (2000 mgm), vitamin A (10,00 IU, unless pregnant), zinc (20 mgm) and pantothenic acid (500 - 1000 mgm) to improve digestive health in general.

Enzyme multi-formulas

A simpler answer may be to take a multi-enzyme preparation. There are several of these on the market. Look for the FCC activity index. This is a far more important guide to the activity of enzymes than weight alone.

Formulas should contain the enzymes required to break down and metabolize the full range of food types. Look for:

- proteases and proteinases (which digest protein)

- lipase (digests fats)

- amylase (digests carbohydrates/starches)

- cellulase, pectinase and phytase (which digest fiber)

- lactase (milk sugar)

- other complex sugar enzymes, such as glucoamylase, invertase, and malt diastase.

- xylanase – breaks down the xylan sugars found in most plants (works well with grains such as corn.

- actinidin – a protease from the kiwi fruit that shows significant activity on wheat products.

Most products will contain bromelain – a broad spectrum enzyme that hydrolizes most soluble proteins, and papain – a proteolytic enzyme characterized by its ability to hydrolyze large proteins into smaller peptides and amino acids. Look out also for Alpha galactosidase, which breaks melibose, raffinose, and stachyose – sugars that are responsible for excess gas in the digestive system.

Malabsorption

It is a mystery to me how serious doctors can acknowledge that food allergy may cause malabsorption syndrome, as in the case of gluten allergy leading to celiac disease, and yet refuse to even *consider* the possibility that other food reactions may do the same, in greater or lesser degree!

My work over the years has made it pretty clear to me that malabsorption is common, almost the norm. This is partly caused by toxins in food, especially those chemicals added to processed foods. Foods are refined and vitiated until they have become quite alien to our digestive system and it would hardly be surprising if functionality suffered a great deal. So it becomes a double-whammy: the foods are nutritionally unsound and then cause malabsorption, leading to further reduction in valuable nutrients. All this taking place, ironically, while the population is growing ever more bloated and obese.

But I know that even sensible foods may also cause this mal-absorption problem. Milk, I think, is notorious in this respect; we are encouraged to swallow milk for its calcium content but it is a paradox I pointed out in my 1993 book *Food Allergy and Environmental Illness* (Thorsons, London, 1993) that the USA, which has the highest dairy intake per capita in the world, also has the highest incidence of osteoporosis. In fact more American women die of fracture of the neck or femur than die of breast cancer, whereas in China, where dairy produce is not a feature of the traditional diet, osteoporosis was virtually unknown (all this may be changing under the onslaught of Western foods).

It follows that one of the major benefits you are going to acquire from my diet program is that you will de-stress your bowel and allow it to recover, eating only safe, healthy foods that are *right for you*. Following the advice of the previous section, you will digest better, reduce bloating, gas emissions, abdominal discomfort and other symptoms, while allowing the whole metabolic process of digestion to place more effectively.

That's one of the reasons people feel wonderful and look great on my program.

Malabsorption tests

Blood tests will help determine whether patients have anemia, low protein levels and deficiencies of certain vitamins and minerals. Blood tests can also be used to make specific diagnoses, for example, anti-endomysial antibody test for celiac disease, which is more sensitive than the older alpha-gliadin antibody test.

Multiple stool studies can be performed to evaluate any patient with malabsorption, particularly when it manifests as diarrhea. Parasites should be excluded as possible causes of malabsorption (competition for nutrients).

Most useful in the evaluation of malabsorption is a fecal fat determination. The patient is asked to ingest at least 80 gm of fat daily, and stools are collected for one to three days. The total amount of fat excreted in the stool is determined in the laboratory. This is helpful in determining the degree of malabsorption; usually less than 7 gm of fat per day are excreted in stool. Bile acid deficiency and bacterial overgrowth usually do not produce fecal fat of more than 30 gm per day. Patients with celiac disease will rarely produce more than 60 gm of fat per day in the stool. Severe steatorrhea (80 - 100 gm of fat per day) is seen in patients with pancreatic insufficiency or in patients who have had large chunks of bowel removed.

The D-xylose test is a very useful test to evaluate the integrity of the intestinal mucosa and its ability to absorb. D-xylose is a sugar that is absorbed across the intestinal mucosa and can be measured in the urine and blood. After a patient drinks the Xylose, urine or blood are collected over the next several hours. Low Xylose levels in the blood or urine are highly suggestive of a abnormality of the intestinal mucosa.

Pancreatic function tests are more elaborate but could add value in difficult cases. A tube is placed through the nose or mouth so that its tip is lying next to the opening of the pancreatic duct into the duodenum. Secretions are collected and the content of bicarbonate and enzymes are measured after the pancreas has been stimulated with a hormone called secretin or with a test meal. Pancreatic insufficiency is indicated if the bicarbonate and enzyme concentrations are very low.

Another pancreatic function test, the Bentiromide test, involves ingestion of a chemical called bentiromide. This is broken down by pancreatic enzymes and one constituent (para-aminobenzoic acid, PABA) is absorbed and excreted in the urine. Pancreatic insufficiency is suspected when urinary PABA levels are low.

[Medical University of South Carolina website: www.ddc.musc.edu/ddc_pub/index.htm

Leaky gut syndrome

Finally, a third model of intestinal health and disease, concerning the way food residues are dealt with by the gut.

It is important to realize that the contents of the bowel are technically outside the body. If you imagine a piece of string entering at the mouth and emerging from the anus, you will readily see this is true. The defined space of the bowel (or lumen) contains a considerable immunological and toxic burden, including potentially allergenic food residues, waste toxins, food toxins (both natural toxins and artificially added man-made chemicals), bacteria, parasites and free radicals released by many processes taking place. Precisely because of our very intimate entanglement with this space, our bodies need to be protected from these deleterious substances.

There is an important barrier mechanism which ensures the danger is contained. The lining of the bowel is designed to be impenetrable to this degraded matter and accepts molecules specially chosen for absorption. There is also an important component of the immune system, right on site in the wall of the intestine, called Peyer's patches. These islands of lymphatic tissue round up and overwhelm suspect immune material, before it breaks free and enters the circulation. At times, this membrane protective layer is overburdened, especially if our lifestyle is abusive, and may let through some of the toxins. These enter the blood in the intestinal network of veins, which is carried straight to the liver, where detoxification takes place.

A serious problem can arise once the impenetrability of the gut mucosa is impaired. We call this "leaky gut syndrome" and a whole cascade of problems can ensue, giving us yet another model of food allergy/ intolerance and toxic overload.

Food as recognizable food gets into the bloodstream and remains identifiable by its immunological source. In other words, "wheat-ness" or "pork-ness" of the food survives. This is then capable of setting up and allergic reaction, to wheat or pork, or whatever culprit is to blame. Even this wouldn't be a problem, if the larger food molecules would only stay put: in the lumen of the bowel.

But they don't.

A vicious circle

As a result of increased permeability, the larger immunologically-active molecules escape into the blood, set up immune complexes, and wreak havoc. This results in an inflammatory process, which can affect all parts of the body, including the gut. This in turn leads to further loss of integrity of the gut wall and further leakage. Thus food allergy can become a cause of the problem, as well as the result, and a kind of vicious circle is entered.

The liver tries to handle these extra-large molecules and remove absorbed toxins, which should have remained behind in the bowel. When this happens the liver is also overloaded, leading to compromise of the cytochrome p-450 detox system (one of the main detox pathways), with resultant escape of toxins, production of excess free radicals and loss of nutritional essentials, such as glutathione and other sulphur-containing amino acids. The liver has to dispose of toxins somewhere and usually this ends up in the bile (most mercury, for example, is excreted into the bile). "Toxic bile" in turn will injure the gut mucosa and a second vicious circle is in progress. Toxic bile is also known to lead to chronic pancreatitis and possible pancreatic cancer [Braganza, J.M., Pancreatic disease: a casualty of hepatic "detoxification"? *Lancet,* 1983. ii: p. 1000-1002].

But it is worse. For every toxic molecule excreted in the bile, the liver has given up one molecule of precious glutathione, to create a conjugate. That is what is supposed to happen. But when the conjugate enters the bowel and encounters more toxic bile with active free radicals, these attack the conjugate and release the toxin once more. The glutathione molecule is wasted and the toxin is back on the loose.

You will see at once why a diet rich in antioxidants is really essential in combating the chemical plague of our world. We cannot go on squandering our biological reserve in this way, without facing increased risk of cancer and, of course, accelerating the ageing process.

Verifying leaky gut syndrome

A neat and useful model. But is it valid? A test has been developed to establish whether or not the gut is releasing larger molecules than are biologically acceptable. It concerns absorption of two complex sugars, mannitol and lactulose.

Mannitol is a relatively small molecule and should be absorbed; lactulose is larger and should not be absorbed significantly. The patient fasts and both sugars are administered simultaneously. The information which can be gained is interesting:

- · If the absorption of mannitol is low, suspect malabsorption.
- · If the absorption of lactulose is high, suspect leaky gut.
- · If both are normal, this suggests healthy gut performance.

In fact what is normally measured is the mannitol/lactulose ratio. A recent study published in the Lancet found that the lactulose-mannitol ratio was an accurate predictor of relapse when measured in patients with Crohn's disease who were clinically in remission (Wyatt, J., et al., Intestinal permeability and the prediction of relapse in Crohn's disease. Lancet, 1993. 341(8858): p. 1437-9).

Improving a leaky gut

Obviously enzyme supplements, as described earlier in this chapter, will assist in overcoming the problem, because more of the immunologically active residues will be reduced to harmless smaller molecules.

Eliminating unsafe foods, using this personalized approach, will also reduce bowel inflammation. So it will tend to improve through time.

Other correctable pathology to look for includes parasites. Giardia, cryptosporidium, worms, amebas and flukes all inflame the gut wall and will tend to create permeability. These are far from rare. Indeed, Dr. William P. Stuppy, a Harvard trained gastroenterologist and pathologist gave a paper at the 2006 Annual Scientific Meeting of The American College of Gastroenterology with some worrying figures. For people with abdominal complaints, even mild, or just fatigue, sleeplessness and vague rashes, he was finding parasites. Lots of 'em.

In fact he found that among 672 patients, they shared a total of 2210 parasite infections. That means some individuals had two or more parasites.

The critters he found were as follows:

Cryptosporidium parvum: 243
Amoeba histolytica: 213
Helicobacter pylori: 212
Giardia lamblia: 163
Clostridium difficile: 114 (related to gangrene and botulism)
Blastocystis hominis: 41
Ascaris lumbricoides, a common and vicious roundworm: 64
Taenia soleum, the pork tapeworm: 32
Trichinella spiralis, the pork tissue worm that literally crawls through
    your body: 23

It is interesting that Cryptosporidium is the commonest and affects 1/3rd of patients. Five percent had the pork tapeworm, which can be pretty gruesome. The first sign some patients have of its presence is a wriggling strap that flops from the anus.

The important point of the study is that it shows that nasty parasites are a common cause in anyone with gastrointestinal complaints that check out negative on endoscopy and all the usual tests. I would add fatigue of all kinds, including Lyme's and fibromyalgia. I used to find lots of these animals in my allergy practice back in the UK. An individual can become allergic to the parasites they are carrying, making the picture sometimes very complex.

Stuppy used a very simple saliva test for estimating parasites load. This technique, run by Diagnos-Techs lab, in Washington, gives an accurate

measure of IgG and IgA antibodies against these varied organisms (www.
diagnos-techs.com). It's non-invasive and does not even require an office
visit. These tests are available through your care provider and are relatively
cheap, compared to blood work and stool samples – though these may also
be recommended to establish a fuller diagnosis.

Just remember my caution about hospital labs and their skills with
a microscope! You would be better to send your samples to a good lab and
I recommend the following:

Institute of Parasitic Diseases
Diagnostic Laboratory
3530 E. Indian School Road, Suite 3
Phoenix, Arizona 85018
602-955-4211

The Director at the Institute of Parasitic Diseases, Dr. Omar M. Amin, was
a Professor of Parasitic Epidemiology at the University of Wisconsin and
currently is Professor of Parasitology at Arizona State University. He has
over one hundred major articles published in journals in human parasitic
infection.

Other labs you might like to consider are as follows:

Genova Diagnostics
18A Regent Park Boulevard
Ashville, North Carolina 28806
800-522-4762

The Center for the Improvement of Human Functioning
3100 North Hillside Ave.
Wichita, Kansas 67219
800-447-7276

Medical Diagnostic Laboratory
3250 Westchester Ave.
Bronx, New York 10461
212-828-1500

What to do?

The first thing I teach patients is that "treatment" is not about killing parasites; that comes into it, but proper treatment is about terrain. If you are a walk-in territory for parasites, you had better fix yourself up so they have a rough time and cannot easily survive. The single biggest item I ever found for terrain problems (applies to Candida too) was heavy metal toxicity. Mercury is the worst offender, of course, but there are others: arsenic, lead (big problem), aluminum and chromium, to name a few. Then comes xenobiotic chemicals, such as benzene, phthalates, toluene and xylene. So parasites are really a mixed message – you've got them but you've also got other problems too.

You need to fix these terrain problems. Meantime get some chlorella, and I urge you to consider "Beyond Chelation" from www.Longevityplus. com. It chelates heavy metals but has many other health benefits, such as prevention of cardiovascular disasters. It thins the blood and prevents clotting as well as heparin or warfarin but without the hazards.

Meanwhile there are a number of recognized holistic alternatives for cleansing parasites. My own favorite is "Natural Cleanse" from Ancient Herbal remedies in the UK. 60 capsules costs £GB22.95 (around $US40).

Ingredients: Green Hull Black Walnut (husks), (Juglans regia L.) Cloves (flower) (Eugenia caryophyllata), Pumpkin Seed (Cucurbita pepo L.), Gentian Root (Gentiana Lutea L.), Hyssop (leaves) (Hyssopus officinalis L.), Black Seed (Nigella sativa), Wild Peppermint Leaves (Mentha x piperita), Thyme Leaf (Thymus Vulgaris L.), Fennel Seed (Foeniculum vulgare), Grapefruit Seed (Citrus paradise Macf.), Oregano (Origanum vulgare).

Natural Cleanse is a 500-year old remedy, well tried and tested to work against parasites. It also has strong anti-fungal properties and is used to assist with the elimination of moulds, fungi and yeasts, including Candida albicans. Acting as a scavenger in the bloodstream, Natural Cleanse uses taste, texture and heat to create an inhospitable environment for parasites to exist. This explains its broad spectrum application for the many different parasite groups. Natural Cleanse is recommended over a minimum four-month period in order to catch parasites in all their stages of development. It is a safe program for adults, children and animals.

To order Natural Cleanse go to www.resourcesforlife.net

You may need colostrum and probiotics, as part of a campaign against dysbiosis. I have discussed this in more detail below. Dr. Stuppy recommends *Saccharomyces boulardii* (250 mgm) and colostrum (960 mgm), by mouth, twice a day, for two weeks. This shifted the organism Clostridium difficile which, as its name implies, is a dog to get rid of.

Specific therapy

In his definitive study, Dr. Stuppy found one treatment, above all others, was over 98% effective against all the above listed pathogens. That was Alinia (generic: nitazoxanide). In fact his hit rate was as follows:

> Cryptosporidium parvum, reduced by 99%,
> Amoeba histolytica, down by 100%,
> Giadria lamblia, 98%
> Blastocystis hominis, 96%
> Ascaris lumbricoides, 90% (difficult one, that)
> Clostridium difficile, down 100%,
> T. solium, 100%
> T. spiralis, 100%

Nitazoxanide is highly effective in treating/eradicating gastrointestinal pathogens; this includes parasites, helminths, protozoa, and pathologic bacteria.

Alinia is available on prescription in the US (around $18 a capsule) but I feel bound to point out you can get the generic compound (nitazoxanide) in Mexico far cheaper!

The dosage Dr. Stuppy used was 1 gram, twice daily, for two weeks. This is heavy medication.

Once cleared, I suggest readers consider using it rather differently, as a "worming pill," just like we do for cats and dogs. Take 1 gram, twice a day, for three days. Repeat every six months. But don't forget to fix the terrain, otherwise the parasites will all come back!

21

Candida and The Human Microbiome

Finally, a topic that is worth a whole book in itself! You may have heard the saying that "death begins in the colon." That may just be a subject for debate, but there is no question that a great deal of bad feeling and ill-health begins in the gut. I say "bad feelings" advisedly because it is evident that our emotions also impact the gut. We have expressions like "gut feeling" for an emotional response, and "I felt a knot in my stomach" or "I nearly crapped my pants" for fear. It works the other way too: if we have bad feelings in the belly we say, "I feel sick."

The fact is that the state of our intestines has a great impact on our general health and well-being. Yet it happens to be one of the most unhealthy terrains in most people.

Food allergy and genetic food intolerance is part of that picture, as we have seen throughout these pages. But there is another big issue which complicates matters a great deal: intestinal infections. We all know there are supposed to be certain bacteria or "germs" in our gut that are friendly and help out with digestion. We call these allies gut "flora," which is really a botanical term. An analogy would be weeds and flowers in the garden: if the beds are crowded with healthy plants, these will choke off weeds before they can become established. But the plants, or "flora," of the gut are supposed to be non-pathogenic, meaning they should not provoke symptoms of disease. Or at least they only do so in special situations, where the body's defenses are weakened, as with AIDs or cancer.

Then a normally harmless organism can run riot and become troublesome, even dangerous. We call this an "opportunistic infection."

One common reason for opportunistic infections is bad diet and bad lifestyle, leading to compromised immunity. An even more important cause is the abuse of antibiotics over the last fifty years. These admittedly remarkable drugs come with a price-tag few doctors take into their reckoning: for every unfriendly bacterium killed there are also friendly ones destroyed. This can have far-reaching and unpleasant consequences for the host organism. As a result the pathogenic species may gain a footing and cause unwanted symptoms and disease.

Food allergy and intolerance is just one of the complications of these opportunistic infections. The intestinal lining becomes damaged and too many foreign substances are absorbed, setting up allergy overload and food chemical reactions, all of which can make the task of tracking down your bad foods and creating a personal safe diet much more difficult.

One such opportunistic organism is *Candida albicans*, the thrush germ, and it is a good starting place for understanding this general upheaval in bowel flora that we call dysbiosis (literally, messed up organisms). You may have read about this infection or heard the term Candidiasis; health magazines and web pages are full of it. But the story is not nearly as simple as untrained or inexperienced writers like to portray.

Let me share with you some real knowledge, acquired over twenty-five years. You will need to know this to be really *Diet Wise* ...

The Candida hypothesis

Dr. Orion Truss of Birmingham, Alabama first brought the candida hypothesis forward in 1978. Dr. Truss is a psychiatrist with a special interest in clinical ecology; his seminal papers in the Journal of Orthomolecular Psychiatry ["Tissue Injury Induced by Candida Albicans," vol. 7, no 1, 1978, pp 17-37 and "Restoration of Immune Competence to Candida Albicans," vol. 9, no 4, 1980, pp 287-301] certainly revealed an extensive and fascinating area of personal investigation. His work was taken up enthusiastically by the late Dr. William Crook, who did more than any single individual to popularize the candida hypotheses, or what has now become known as 'the yeast connection,' taken from the title of his book. [*The Yeast Connection*, Professional Books, 1983].

Since that time, the whole theory seems to have gripped the public's imagination and clinical ecologists have been keen to extol the existence of the problem and the enormous benefits to be gained from tackling it vigorously. The fact is there are health gains to be made by following a so-called anti-Candida program, taking antifungal drugs and excluding sugar and yeast foods from one's diet. Yet Truss's idea is no more than a theory. Please remember that.

Historical background

Truss was in fact far from being the first investigator in this field. My late British colleague Dr. Keith Eaton researched this topic extensively and found Truss's ideas were anticipated almost seventy years earlier by a physician called Turner, who presented a paper on what he termed 'intestinal germ carbohydrate fermentation' [Proceedings of the Royal Society of Medicine Symposium of Intestinal Toxaemia, 1911] [Eaton KK, Gut fermentation: a reappraisal of an old clinical condition with diagnostic tests and management: discussion paper, J Roy Soc Med 1991; 84: 669-71].

In 1931 Arthur F. Hurst was in his footsteps, writing about 'intestinal carbohydrate dyspepsia' [Hurst AF, Knott FA, Intestinal carbohydrate dyspepsia, Quart J Med 1930-31; 24: 171-80]. In the 1930s and 1940s this dyspepsia was being treated with *Lactobacillus acidophilus*, B vitamin supplements and a low-starch diet (remarkably like modern anti-candida treatment except that legumes are no longer banned, as they were at that time).

Medical literature has tried to define the patient-type who suffers with this syndrome. A major text on gastroenterology in 1976 described victims as "*Essentially unhappy people... any suggested panacea or therapeutic straw is grasped... no regime is too severe and no programme [sic] too difficult... with the tenacity of the faithful, they grope their way from one practitioner to the next in the search for a permanently successful remedy.*" This disparaging description shows a lamentable weakness on the part of doctors for blaming any patient they cannot help.

The 'problem patient' attitude was probably what sank the condition in the 1950s. At that time, the psychosomatic theory of disease was enjoying a great revival. The tendency was to dismiss all patients with vague, ill-defined symptoms as psychiatric cases. Unlike today, there were no physical findings to disprove the psychiatric label and so it stuck. It's still with us, to a large degree.

Intestinal fermentation

So the idea of a yeast-like gut pathogen that lives on starches and sugars and causes bowel disturbance is far from new. It seems to enjoy a vogue in medical circles every few decades and then lapses out of sight once again. The reason is probably that, as in the 1980s, some doctors become convinced they know what causes the syndrome, but then can't seem to find a workable proof that affords a satisfactory explanation. This casts doubt on the basis of the theory. So it is today with 'Candida.'

One thing is certain, there is virtually no correlation between Candida in the stool sample and the existence of the 'yeast syndrome.' Indeed, *Candida albicans* is rarely identified in specimens, despite its known very wide occurrence. This lack of correlation is disappointing but hardly surprising, especially if we are looking for the wrong culprit.

It is true that treatment directed towards this type of organism can be highly effective in selected individuals, so clearly a real phenomenon exists. But that doesn't prove that Candida is the true culprit and I want to make sure readers do not fall into this logical trap. In fact I'd like to set the debate alight with the claim that the culprit may not be Candida at all, or that Candida is only one of many potential suspects.

Other available flora that might be at work include the yeasts of the genus *Saccharomyces* (food yeasts), many different types of bacteria, viruses, protozoa, parasites and other strange organisms called archea. In fact I would like to suggest this whole thing is never just one organism, but many.

On-board brewery

Historically, *Sarcina ventriculata* is an important organism. In the old days, when surgeons operated in top hats and frock coats, often smoking a cigar while they butchered, once in a while they would literally blow up their patients as the alcoholic gases generated by Sarcina were released from the patient's stomach when cut open; the cigar would ignite the fumes and a fireball was the disastrous result!

These 'on-board breweries' are probably quite common. In the early 80s we began to realize that an individual could present with quite high levels of blood alcohol and yet be a non-drinker. There have been several celebrated cases, including one of my own, in which individuals who were guilty of driving under the influence of alcohol were able to show they had not been drinking but that they did have significant infections with Candida and so escaped the laws.

It may help to do a carbohydrate fermentation test: to fast, followed by a challenge dose of fermentable sugars, and serial blood tests. This will show if the sugars are being fermented or not.

But just as Candida isn't the only contender for the role of pathogen, ordinary ethyl alcohol is not the only product of biological fermentation we seem to be dealing with. Many other substances can be derived from the breakdown of sugars and starches, including tartaric acid and short-chain fatty acids such as acetate, proprionate, succinate and butyrate, and other alcohols such as iso-propanol, butanol and 2,3-butylene glycol. Testing for these substances is now available commercially in certain centers and may provide useful insights.

Of course it is not just about what the body produces on board but the further fate of these compounds. Such substances should be swiftly eliminated by the detoxification process. But if detoxification pathways are blocked due to overload, many other non-alcohol but equally unwanted metabolites will accumulate, such as epoxides, aldehydes and even chloral hydrate, the potent ingredient of the classic 'Mickey Finn'. Typically this chemical produces a tired and 'spacey' feeling. Here is at least part of the reason these patients can't take alcoholic drinks.

The hydrogen breath test will also reveal compounds in exhaled air which can give a clue to the state of bowel flora.

Breath hydrogen test

In Man, only anaerobic bacteria in the colon are capable of producing hydrogen in our bodies. They do this by fermenting sugars, such as lactose, sucrose, sorbitol, fructose, lactulose etc. (depending on the purpose of the test). The hydrogen enters the bloodstream and is out-gassed via the lungs. This gives rise to the possibility of testing breath for hydrogen content as a means of estimating bacterial activity in the colon.

Prior to hydrogen breath testing, individuals fast for at least twelve hours. At the start of the test, the individual blows into a balloon, filling the balloon. The concentration of hydrogen is measured in a sample of breath removed from the balloon. The individual then ingests a small amount of the test sugar. Additional breath samples are collected and analyzed for hydrogen every fifteen minutes for three to five hours.

Any significant production of hydrogen means that there has been a problem with digestion or absorption of the test sugar and that some of the sugar has reached the colon.

When rapid intestinal transit is present, the test dose of non-digestible lactulose reaches the colon more quickly than normal, and, therefore, hydrogen is produced by the colonic bacteria soon after the sugar is ingested. When bacterial overgrowth of the small bowel is present, ingestion of lactulose results in two separate periods during the test in which hydrogen is produced, an earlier period caused by the bacteria in the small intestine and a later one caused by the bacteria in the colon.

The short-chain fatty acids in the stool and urinary metabolite panel also referred to should help in firmly establishing that something is definitely wrong.

The problem with Candida diets

Candida was really just a hook to hang things on. Do not believe what you read in the media and on the Web, unless the author specifically acknowledges this lack of real understanding. I will attempt to summarize just what we do know about so-called Candida and dysbiosis and also put an end to some of the nonsense and falsehoods, spread principally by unqualified medical practitioners. Many of these enthusiastic amateurs have set themselves up as 'Candida experts' and are making belligerent claims they cannot justify and treating individuals with techniques that are sometimes worthless or – at worst – downright dangerous.

Some of the confusion about Candida comes from the fact that a number of widely circulated 'anti-candida diets' do have beneficial effects, at least at first. What isn't understood is that the mechanism at work is often that of eliminating a food allergy and not eradicating the candida at all. I saw one diet in Sweden which asked patients to exclude dairy produce as part of an anti-Candida regime; a naturopath in Britain says 'no grains.' There is absolutely no rationale for these omissions in the fight against Candida, but these methods ensure that a great many people who are dairy or wheat allergic will 'miraculously' get better. This creates the false impression that the patients did indeed have Candida.

Another incorrect datum that has gained much currency is that once you have Candida you are stuck with it. One hears of people who are supposed to have had it for years. Again, the amateur meddlers' fundamental lack of knowledge is to blame. Because they are not able to prescribe proper antifungal drugs – and indeed, to protect their own shaky position as unlicensed 'experts' some even say that it is undesirable to take antifungals – they are not able to effect proper eradication. This means that many sufferers are denied the full treatment that they need, treatment that would enable them to overcome their condition.

Patients also add to the confusion. Many times I have been confronted with an individual who claimed that every time they ate a certain food, the "Candida" ran riot and swept through their bodies within minutes.

This is really just another subjective symptom of the kind I described in Chapter 10, but often nothing would dissuade them from their own interpretation of events. The trouble magnifies when such individuals go on to write articles or even, God forbid, a book about Candida!

Because of the confusion I have described, I will use the terms Candida, yeast syndrome and intestinal fermentation syndrome interchangeably in the remainder of this chapter. But we must bear in mind the bacterial component also. The whole issue of disordered bowel flora should be referred to simply as dysbiosis or, as we shall soon learn, disordered microbiome.

Testing for Candida and yeasts

I used to carry out a kind of intradermal testing known as provocation-neutralization, or Miller's method. It soon became obvious to me that skin tests for Candida (Oidium, as we used to call it) were of little worth – but testing for yeast was helpful; I used to test baker's yeast and brewer's yeast separately.

Nothing really beats a detailed case history and carefully documenting symptoms. For instance, chemical sensitivity seems to go almost hand in hand with dysbiosis and one may be leading to the other. Conversely, dealing effectively with one would relieve the other. This is knowledge you can't find in books; it's just picked up in clinical experience, from tens of thousands of cases.

There are four symptoms in all that I have found very helpful in pinpointing candida, yeast overgrowth and other causes of dysbiosis:

1.   a craving for sweet foods
2.   a poor tolerance of alcohol
3.   chemical sensitivity
4.   abdominal bloating.

This is my 'awesome four-some'! All four symptoms means almost a certainty; any three will do for a strong presumptive diagnosis. Craving for sugary foods is often outstanding.

You can ask for the fasting glucose alcohol challenge test and breath hydrogen test, as I have described above.

The moldy patient

I continue to use the concept of "Candida" in talking to patients since most people have heard of it and believe that is what they have. However, I prefer the flippant label I used in my *Allergy Handbook* (Thorsons, 1988), the so-called 'moldy patient.' It is a term that stays in the mind, broadens out the debate and gives better insight into what we are dealing with. Whatever the nature of this illness, its manifestation is of a disease caused by encountering and being sensitized by biological products from yeasts, fungi and molds.

Patients are made worse by anything that can be fermented, such as starch and sugars; they react to foodstuffs containing yeast or mold (bread, wine, mushrooms etc.); they are often ill in moldy or musty surroundings (old buildings, woodlands or animal byres); some are even sensitive to damp weather, when molds are sporing freely; often there are accompanying infections of the fungus type, including athlete's foot or other skin infections such as Tinea and Epidermophyton.

Finally, the patient may have been diagnosed as having Thrush, either in the mouth, gut or vagina, which is indisputably caused by the organism *Candida albicans*.

Treatment spectrum

Treatment is really a spectrum, not just one action. Taking antifungal medications is not enough and may not even be needed, if you follow the rest of this advice.

The secret to success, as you have learned all the way through this book, is lowering the body burden. That means cutting molds and yeast out of your diet, at least short-term. But you must also eradicate fermentable foods, otherwise it is like taking with one hand and giving with the other. If you reduce fermentable foods, notably sugars and starches, you starve the enemy into submission. A supply blockade is one of the oldest military tactics in the book!

Use non-fermentable sweeteners if you must, like sorbitol and xylitol, but please NOT aspartame or sucralose (see page XXX)!

Extreme denials are not called for. Some writers foolishly recommend avoidance of fruit and similar natural foods. Others say no root vegetables because the soil in which they grow contains many molds! This may lead to dangerous inadequacies in nutrition and is bad advice because it isn't necessary. Anyone with 'Candida' made ill by eating fruit has a fruit allergy, almost certainly. Those who feel unwell after eating sugars may really have a degree of carbohydrate intolerance due to deficient enzymes.

In the appendix, there is a comprehensive review of yeast and yeast-related food contacts that you should avoid, some of them strictly, some of them as far as possible.

A Note About Mushrooms and Fungi

We all continue to learn and get smarter as we get older (I hope!) So it is that I have learned the helpful anti-Candida, anti-mold, properties of certain mushrooms and fungi.

I used to ban these foods routinely on an anti-Candida program, based on their relationship with yeasts. In fact, biologically, they are not closely related at all but come from a different classification "Kingdom".

Moreover, mushrooms and fungi contain powerful immune boosters called beta-glucans. Some of these are so strong, they have been tapped and used for anti-cancer treatments. Mushrooms known to have great immune-booster properties include shiitake (common in most supermarkets), Reishi (*Ganoderma lucidum*), Maitake (sometimes called "hen of the woods") and turkey-tail mushroom.

Rather than banning these foods, I now actively encourage patients to eat them. Easting mushrooms brings variety and relief to a strict exclusion regime and, I now believe, is very supportive to those battling so-called "yeast syndrome".

Antifungals

Next comes consideration of antifungal medications. Specific drugs described here must be prescribed by a competent physician. Nystatin was the one which started us out and is still going strong (N.Y. STATe INstitute of Chemists). Even among allergics it is well tolerated. The usual doses are in the range of 1,000,000 units = quarter of a teaspoon, four times daily.

Remember: Nystatin can act as a chelating agent (that is, it binds to metals and blocks them) and so should not be taken with nutritional supplements (it would remove zinc, magnesium etc.).

Alternatives include ketoconazole (Nizoral) tablets and fluconazole (Diflucan) capsules. The latter is expensive but easy to take. A 'one-shot' form exists, for those likely to develop reactions to medication. Except for Nystatin, lengthy treatments should not be undertaken, as side-effects are potentially serious, particularly liver toxicity.

Much is disseminated about the 'burn off' reaction patients sometimes get when first starting antifungal treatment. This is similar to the Herxeimer reaction that syphilis patients used to get when starting a course of penicillin; it was caused by a flood of circulating dead spirochetes (syphilis germs). Burn-off (a sudden exacerbation of symptoms) does exist but is much exaggerated and rarely amounts to anything serious. Temporary discontinuance allows it to settle and, nine times out of ten, when the patient resumes the treatment there is no further trouble.

Caprylic Acid

Caprylic acid (a medium-chain triglyceride) is an anti-fungal agent found naturally in coconuts. It smells and tastes horrible but it well known for its anti-Candida properties. It's sometimes called octanoic acid.

Caprylic acid is a commerical antimicrobial pesticide used as a food contact surface sanitizer in commercial food handling establishments on dairy equipment, food processing equipment, breweries, wineries, and beverage processing plants. It is also used as disinfectant in health care facilities, schools/colleges, animal care/veterinary facilities, industrial facilities, office buildings, recreational facilities, retail and wholesale establishments, livestock premises, restaurants, and hotels/motels. In addition, caprylic acid is used as an algaecide, bactericide, and fungicide in nurseries, greenhouses, garden centers, and interiorscapes on ornamentals.

Capricin, a trade brand of caprylic acid, has been frequently advocated as an antifungal. Like malic acid in the vagina, it creates a hostile environment for pathogens. Caprylic acid is the active ingredient in a new medical food validated by scientific research as an effective treatment for Alzheimer's. The medical food is being marketed under the name Axona.

Now The Real Story

OK, that was the story, as it was known, up until about 1995. Since then, things have got steadily more interesting, more complex and actually more understandable.

Let me introduce you to the human microbiome. You will recognize the term biome from the discovery of our own (human) genome. This is the collection of DNA that is supposed to code for "human-ness", though cracks are already beginning to appear in that story.

What we already know is that nobody, and I mean nobody, has the human genome. In fact there is no such thing as the "real" human genome. We are all different and vary by tiny little alterations in the code called single-nucleotide polymorphisms or SNPs (we pronounce "snips"). These small variations are not enough to grow three legs or two heads. But they can easily mean that an individual may not be able to metabolize a particular food safely.

This is a whole new take on what we once called "food allergies". We clinicians were right: there is a food reaction. But the model of how this occurs has shifted somewhat towards metabolic intolerance interpretation, rather than an immune reaction.

OK so far?

Well, now it really shifts gear! In just the last decade we have begun to realize that our gut flora actually contributes more to our genome than we do. About a hundred times more, in fact. This is new and a total shock.

Collectively, the organisms in our gut add up to several trillion microbes. There are probably over 1,000 species living in and travelling on "Planet Human". They too have genetic coding, albeit simple.

This is called the (human) microbiome and it has just as much impact on our food tolerances as our own genes and SNPs. Not surprisingly, really, since they are thousands of times more microbial genes in the pool than human genes.

It has been a total shock and yet wonderfully revealing and liberating. At last I begin to understand all those effects that were so clear to me, in a clinical setting, almost forty years ago.

Why Is This Important?

Fascinating? Yes. Incredible, even. But why is it so important? Because the microbiome regulates our immune system in ways we could not have guessed a quarter century ago.

We are born sterile, of course. The womb has no microbes. But during the process of birth Momma infects us with her shit (call it "fecal organisms" if you can't handle that vulgar word). It's the most wonderful gift to her child. Because of it, the baby's immune system comes into contact with typical human flora. It is educated by contact.

We now realize this education process is more than just a good idea; it's essential and if it doesn't happen in an orderly way—and to the right organisms—the baby gets off on completely the wrong foot and... guess what? It suffers with food allergies, rashes, atopic disease, rhinitis, ear infections, all the usual stuff which results when the immune system is not performing properly.

In mice kept sterile of microbes, immune tissue fails to mature properly and carries fewer of the signaling molecules that sense and react to pathogens. The immune system does not perform properly, as it should.

Once again Nature has confounded us with her simple wisdom. Moms and doctors running around with antiseptic wipes and bottles of disinfectant have misunderstood the issues completely. We need our germs. They live with us; they help us; they are us!

We need healthy bowel flora, like we need food and oxygen. Disordered bowel flora or dysbiosis is a serious disease. It means ill health in spades. It means our human-ness is lost. No wonder then, that blasting it all to ruin with broad-spectrum antibiotics means there is a price to pay.

So now you are really "Diet Wise"!

Probiotics

This is where probiotics come in. In a nutshell; we need to get our bowel flora back to healthy and fast. That means more than just removing the offenders and re-colonization with suitable, friendly flora.

It means we have to re-grow our entire gut garden. Just like a gardener, we have to pull weeds, plant good crops, feed and nurture those crops till they flourish and avoid the factors which favor weeds.

In other words, we change our diet, to avoid sugars and junk; get decent fresh and natural foods to eat; we replace the unfriendly microbes with more suitable ones: our own bacterial friends and allies.

Most well known among these friendly bacteria is Lactobacillus acidophilus, the yoghurt-making germ. Many supplements of 'acidophilus' are currently being marketed. Some contain very few live bacteria and are of poor value, if not completely fraudulent.

In fact Bifidobacteria and Bacteroides are much more prevalent in the gut; both are anaerobic, comprising some ninety percent of natural bowel flora and as much as two thirds of the weight of faeces. Top brand "probiotics", as these flora supplements are known, now include primarily Bifidobacteria. Look for those that provide human-strain acidophilus; logically these are more likely to establish themselves in the human colon.

The NCFM strain of Lactobacillus is favored currently, because of its ability to survive stomach acid after ingestion and is chosen for whole-genome sequencing, which contains 1,864 predicted protein-encoding genes, including human-friendly enzymes. This is a measure of how much and how fast nutrigenomics is taking over in the field of healthy diet. The NCFM strain has been used safely for over twenty-five years and there is scientific evidence it can modulate immune activity. [Appl Environ Microbiol. 2005 August; 71(8): 4925–4929. doi: 10.1128/AEM.71.8.4925-4929.2005.]

One important point: whichever preparation you buy, please remember that pill manufacture, a process which crushes the organisms, naturally kills most of the viable bacteria. Choose a supply from a manufacturer who makes a point of preventing this destructive occurrence.

Finally, please remember: just swallowing probiotics and doing nothing else is no more a sensible approach to health than taking pills and medicines. It's a whole-body act of eating well, good lifestyle, wise choices and gradually building back the damaged microbiome.

Other probiotics you might consider include these:

Sauerkraut (fermented cabbage) contains the beneficial microbes leuconostoc, pediococcus, and lactobacillus. Choose unpasteurized sauerkraut because pasteurization (used to treat most supermarket sauerkraut) kills active, beneficial bacteria. Sauerkraut -- and the similar but spicy Korean dish, kimchi -- is also loaded with immune-boosting vitamins that may help ward off infection.

Miso: a popular breakfast food in Japan, this fermented soybean paste really can get your digestive system moving. Probiotic-filled miso reportedly contains more than 160 bacteria strains. It's often used to make a salty soup that is low in calories and high in B vitamins and protective antioxidants.

Tempeh could work. Made from a base of fermented soybeans, this Indonesian patty produces a type of natural antibiotic that fights certain bacteria. In addition, tempeh is very high in protein. Its flavor has often been described as smoky, nutty, and similar to a mushroom. Tempeh can be marinated and used in meals in place of meat.

Pre-Biotics

While probiotic-foods contain live bacteria, prebiotic foods feed the good bacteria already living in your digestive system. Pre-biotics are mainly fiber-based foods, that provide a matrix in which probiotics can grow.

You can find prebiotics in foods such as asparagus, Jerusalem artichokes, bananas, oatmeal, red wine, honey, maple syrup, and legumes. Consider eating pre-biotic foods on their own or with probiotic foods, to perhaps give the probiotics a boost.

Also consider adding to the diet fructo-oligosaccharides (FOS), which act as a food source to nourish healthful bacteria but not unhealthful ones. FOS is extracted from fruits and vegetables such as bananas, onions, chicory root, garlic, asparagus, barley, wheat, jícama, and leeks. Some grains and cereals, such as wheat, also contain amounts of FOS. The Jerusalem artichoke and its relative yacón have been found to have the highest concentrations of FOS of cultured plants.

Thank you for your determination and persistence in reading this far and I wish you the very best in your pursuit of health, happiness and longevity.

**For more information on health topics in general,
be sure to visit my website:
www.alternative-doctor.com**

Appendix A

Food Families

This appendix gives a list of food families and also foods without commonly eaten relatives. Use this as a guide in making up your own rotation diet.

There is a great deal of cross-reacting between different members of a food family. However, this does not mean that if you are allergic to one food all other members of that same family need be condemned. For example, it is possible to be violently allergic to potato but OK with tomato. This *does* mean, however, that you should be more suspicious of related foods.

Note that ham and bacon belong with pork, dairy produce with beef, and eggs with chicken. Once again, though, it doesn't follow automatically that you will be allergic to all products from a certain animal. It is possible to be very allergic to milk and dairy produce and yet be (reasonably) safe with beef.

Study the table carefully; it will repay your effort.

THE PLANT KINGDOM

Apple family: apple, pear, quince, medlar (crabapple)
Avocado family: avocado, cinnamon, sassafras
Banana family: banana, arrowroot, plantain
Beechnut family: beechnut, chestnut, black pepper
Blueberry family: blueberry (various names), cranberry, wintergreen
Buckwheat family: buckwheat, rhubarb
Carrot family: carrot, celery, parsnip, parsley, dill, fennel, anise, caraway, cumin, coriander
Cashew family: cashew, pistachio, mango, chicle (principle ingredient of chewing gum)
Chinese artichoke
Citrus family: orange, grapefruit, lemon, lime, tangerine, citron, kumquat, clementine (a small, sweet variety of tangerine with orange-red skin), ugli (a large, sweet variety of tangelo)
Coffee
Cola family: chocolate, cola, karaya gum (used as a thickening agent in cosmetics and foodstuffs)

Composite family: lettuce, endive, chicory, globe artichoke, Jerusalem artichoke, sunflower, dandelion, chamomile, goldenrod, safflower

Crucifer family: cabbage, Brussels sprouts, broccoli, cauliflower, kale, collards, kohlrabi, mustard, turnip, rutabaga, swede, rape, horseradish, Chinese cabbage, watercress

Elderberry

Ginger family: ginger, turmeric, ginseng

Gooseberry family (saxifrages): gooseberry, black currant, red currant

Grape family: grape, muscatel (muscat grape), raisins, sultanas (a small, seedless raisin) [note: 'currants' are dried grapes]

Grass family: bamboo, barley, wheat, rye, oats, rice, millet, sugar cane, sorghum, corn

Guava family: guava, allspice, clove, gum acacia

Lily family: garlic, onion, shallot, leek, chives, asparagus

Lychee nut

Macadamia nut

Maple sugar

Mint family: peppermint, spearmint, horsemint (also called wild bergamot), water mint, basil, lavender oil, rosemary, marjoram, sage, horehound, savory, thyme

Mulberry family: mulberry, figs, breadfruit

Mushrooms, fungi

Nightshade family: tomato, potato, eggplant, tobacco, green and red peppers, capsicum

Nutmeg family: nutmeg, mace

Okra family: okra (bindi), cottonseed

Palm family: coconut, sago, date, Taro, poi

Papaya

Persimmon

Pineapple

Plum family: plum, prune, peach, apricot, almond, cherry, greengage

Pulses (legumes) *family:* peanut, pea, beans, lentils, licorice, gum tragancanth, quinoa, sarsaparilla

Spinach family: spinach, chard, beetroot, sugar beet

Squashe family: melon, watermelon, pumpkin, squash, cucumber, zucchini, marrow squash

Strawberry family: strawberry, raspberry, blackberry

Sweet potato

Tapioca

Tea

Vanilla

Walnut family: walnut, pecan, hickory, Water chestnuts

THE ANIMAL KINGDOM

Sea Food
Anchovy
Bass, mullet, grouper
Butterfish
Carp
Catfish
Cetaceae; whale, dolphin (these are, of course, mammals)
Cod, haddock, hake, coley, whiting
Conger eel
Crustacea: shrimp, lobster, crayfish, crab,
Eel
Fish (there are many families here, which make a confusing array. Only the
    main fishes and groups are included):
Sturgeons
Flounder, turbot, halibut, plaice, dab, sole
Grunt
Herring, pilchards, sprats, shad
Mackerel, tuna, bonito
Molluscs: (Pelecypods) clam, oyster, mussel, scallop; (Gastropods)
snail, conch, abalone; (Cephalopods) squid, octopus
Pike
Puffer
Red snapper
Salmon, trout
Yellow perch, walleye pike

Amphibia
Frog

Reptiles
Turtle, snake, alligator

Birds
Duck family: duck, goose
Eggs: all pretty similar, but experiment. Egg white is usually the most
    allergenic
Grouse family: grouse, turkey, guinea fowl

Pheasant family: chicken, pheasant, quail, partridge, prairie chicken, peafowl, pigeon, snipe, woodcock

Mammals
Cattle: cow, sheep, lamb, mutton, goat, buffalo
Deer: venison, elk, moose, caribou, reindeer
Horse
Lion, tiger
Pig: pork, ham, bacon, gammon
Rabbit family: rabbit, hare
Rodents: domestic guinea pig
Seal

Appendix B

Food Contacts Lists

Patients often find it helpful to have lists of all the possible foods and drinks in which banned (allergenic) substances might be found. Here is a starter list, but I do encourage patients to use their resourcefulness, as there are bound to be omissions. The doctor cannot always be present to watch what is being eaten; it is the patient who needs to have control and a full understanding of all the data available.

Keep in mind that food manufacturing techniques change, ingredients are altered as market forces come into play and items differ from one country or ethnic group to another.

Use these lists as a guide until you get the hang of what to look for.

Remember: not all types of food listed *always* contain a specified ingredient. Often items are listed that simply *may* do so. If there is any real doubt, contact the manufacturers and ask.

Individuals vary. It is sometimes possible to eat a food in some forms but not in others. Thus a certain amount of experimentation is called for.

Where non-edible food contacts are interesting, I have supplied hints concerning these also.

Wheat Contacts

Beverages: beer, gin, whiskies, (in fact any drink containing neutral spirits, malted foods and drinks, such as malted milk, *Ovaltine, Postum*

Breads: white bread, whole-wheat bread, rye bread, hot breads, multi-flour breads (such as German cornbread), rusk, biscuits, muffins, popovers, pretzels, rolls and any foods made with batter (such as waffles, pancakes and crackers)

Cereals: bran flakes, corn flakes (often), *Wheaties, Grape Nuts, Puffed Wheat, Cocoa Puffs, Frosted Flakes, Rice Crispies, Shredded Wheat* and other malted cereals (such as barley malt), farina, wheat germ

Flours: corn flour, gluten-free flour, rice flour, rye flour, white flour, whole-wheat flour. One should not overlook mixtures with wheat flour in

them

Meat, Eggs or Cheese: casseroles, croquettes, timbales, meat loaf, meat patties, hamburgers that include bread, flour or breadcrumbs as ingredients, sausage, wieners, cold cuts, soufflés, meat and fish rolled in flour (Swiss steak)

Pastries and Desserts: cakes, cookies, doughnuts, pies, pastries, puddings, ice cream cones, ice cream (thickening), bread pudding

Potatoes or Substitute/Pastas: scalloped floured potatoes, packaged creamed potatoes, macaroni, noodles, vermicelli, spaghetti, any pasta, dumplings, soufflés and any casseroles or puddings that include flour, bread or breadcrumbs as ingredients

Soups: bouillon cubes, all cream soups thickened with flour, any canned cream soups

Sweets: candy bars, chocolate drink – all chocolate (except bitter cocoa and bitter chocolate)

Vegetables: scalloped tomato, fried vegetables (if floured or breaded), vegetable soufflés, casseroles or puddings including flour, bread or breadcrumbs as ingredients

Miscellaneous: breaded foods, mixtures containing breadcrumbs, flour or bread, mayonnaise (check the label), malted products, gravies, sauces, any fat used for frying food with wheat in it, foods rolled in flour or breadcrumbs and pancake mixtures

Corn Contacts

Note: Maize is the same as corn

Baking: corn flour, corn starch, non-specified flours, stock cubes, tinned and packet soups, batters, baking mixes, doughs, baking powder, gravy mixes, corn oil, any non-specified vegetable oil, confectioner's sugar, jellies, glucose syrup, grits, monosodium glutamate

Beverages: beers, ales, lager, spirits, colas, cordials, lemonade, *Lucozade,* most carbonated soft drinks (they use corn syrup as a sweetener), instant coffee, instant tea

Breads: bread, cornbread, polenta, pizza, pasta, tortilla

Cereals: cornflakes, sugared cornflakes, e.g. *Frosted Flakes*

Confectionery: cakes, cookies, muffins, waffles

Dairy: instant desserts, *Delight,* custard powder, blancmange, branded yoghurts, ice cream, margarine, dairy-free margarine, processed cheeses, soya milk

Drugs and Medicines: aspirin, paracetamol and all white pills and *most* other tablets, syrups, liquid medicines, suppositories, lozenges, capsules, some vitamin pills

Jams, *etc.:* jam, peanut butter, sandwich spreads, canned meat spreads

Meats: sausage, ham, bacon, wurst, variety meats, bolognas, frankfurters; some meats are injected with dextrose to 'sweeten' them

Sauces: ketchup, *OK,* mayonnaise, French dressing, gravy mixes, vinegar, pickles

Sweets: popcorn, chocolate, chocolate 'flavor,' chewing gum, sherbet, glucose tablets, any dextrose-containing food, candy, or zest drink.

Miscellaneous: paper cups, cartons for fruit juice, milk, etc., envelope gum, stamp gum in some countries, sticky labels, talcum powder, tooth-paste and dentifrices, clothing starch, plastic food wrappers (may be coated with corn starch), some wines (may appear on labels as 'modified starch'), etc.

Tip: On a corn-free diet you should avoid all manufactured foods, then it's easy!

Yeasts, Molds and Ferments Contacts

Definition: any substance derived from, cross-reactive with or containing either substantial or trace amount of yeasts (sometimes called leavening), molds (also called fungi), ferments (process of souring, fermentation, fermentation hydrolysis)

All Cheeses: including fermented dairy products, cottage cheese, natural, blended and pasteurized cheeses and sour cream

All Fermented Beverages: beer, wine, champagne, whiskies, rum, brandies, tequila, root beer, ginger ales, as well as all substances that contain alcohol: extracts, tinctures, cough syrups and other medications

All Malted Products: milk drinks that have been malted, sweets that have been malted, malted breakfast cereals

All Raised Doughs: breads, buns, rolls, prepared 'icebox' or frozen breads, some biscuits and crispbreads

All Vinegars: apple, distilled, wine, grape, pear, etc. This includes all foods containing any vinegar, e.g. salad dressings, mayonnaise substitutes, pickles, catsup, sauerkraut, olives, most condiments, sauces (barbecue, tomato, chili, green pepper), mince pie preparations and many others

Antibiotics: penicillin, Amoxycillin, and many other '-illins,' 'Mycin' drugs and related compounds such as Erythromycin, Streptomycin, Chloramphenicol. Tetracyclines and related derivatives: all the cephalosporin derivatives and all others derived from molds and mold cultures

Cereals: those fortified with added vitamins such as thiamin, niacin, riboflavin, etc.

Dried Fruits: prunes, raisins, dates, figs, apricots, etc. Again, some batches may be mold-free but others will have commercially acceptable amounts of mold on the fruit while drying.

Ferments and Molds: soya sauce, pickles etc., truffles, mushrooms

Flours: those that have been 'enriched' (i.e. most flours)

Juices: fruit juices – canned or frozen. (In commercial preparation the *whole* fruit is used, some of which may be moldy but not sufficiently so to be considered spoiled); fresh, home-squeezed should be yeast-free

Milks: if enriched or fortified with vitamins

Vitamins: B, B complex and multiple vitamins containing B complex. Products containing B_6, B_{12} irradiatec ergosterol (vitamin D); all products containing brewer's yeast or derivative

Milk Contacts

Beverages: milk, cream, chocolate or coco drink mixes, cocoa made with milk

Breads: any bread made with milk, milk solids, butter, margarines (check labels)

Cereals: any cooked cereal or mush prepared with milk or cream

Desserts: puddings made with milk, whipped cream toppings, ice cream and sherbet, cake, cookies, prepared flour mixes, pudding mixes, custard
Fats: butter, margarine churned in milk

Meat, Eggs or Cheese: scrambled egg made with milk or prepared in butter or margarine; any meat or fish seared or fried in butter or margarine; all cheeses (au gratin); cold cuts; packaged mixed dishes

Potatoes or Substitute: creamed or scalloped potatoes, gravy, any vegetable seasoned with butter, margarine, milk, cream, cheese (au gratin)

Soups: cream soups made with milk, cream, butter, margarine; all canned cream soups

Sweets: all sweets except plain sugar candy

Vegetables: creamed vegetables, any vegetable seasoned with butter, margarine, milk, cream, cheese

Miscellaneous: creamed foods, boiled salad dressing, white sauces. Read labels on all prepared foods

Soya Contacts

Bakery Goods: soybean flour containing only 1 per cent oil is now used by many bakers in dough mixtures for breads, rolls, cakes and pastries. This keeps them moist and saleable several days longer. Roasted soya nuts are also sometimes used in place of peanuts

Cereals: soy flakes, soya bran

Cheese Substitutes: Tofu, vegetarian cheeses (some), miso
Low-fat Spreads and Butter Substitutes: margarines, etc.; shortening

Meats: sausages, wurst, bologna, saveloy, luncheon meat

Milk Substitutes: soya milk, *Wysoy* (Wyeth), soya ice cream. Some bakeries use soy milk instead of cow's milk

Nuts: soya beans may be roasted and salted and used instead of peanuts

Pastas: soybean noodles, macaroni, spaghetti

Salad Dressings: many of the salad dressings and mayonnaises contain soy oil but only state on the label that they contain vegetable oil. Present conditions have necessitated the use of soy oil in many brands of oil previously free of soybean

Sauces: ketchup, OK sauce (brown sauce), *Kitchen Bouquet,* soya sauce, *Lea & Perrins,* Worcester sauce (any)

Sweets: soya flour is used in hard candies, nut candies, and caramels. Lecithin is invariably derived from soybean and is used in candies to prevent drying out and to emulsify the fats

Miscellaneous: varnish, paints, enamels, printing ink, candles, celluloid, cloth, massage creams, linoleum, paper sizing, adhesives, fertilizer, nitroglycerine, paper finishes, blankets, soap, fish food, custards, fodder, glycerine, textile dressings, lubricating oil, illuminating oil

Appendix C

Seven-Day Stone Age Diet

Suggested menus and recipes

Many people, I know from experience, would like to try the Stone Age diet but find it daunting. It is something of a revolution. I have joked with patients on many occasions that they must change their shopping habits, never mind eating habits!

Here are some suggestions for those of you who want to know how to go about it. My nurse Marion Whiting went to the trouble of working out a seven-day menu plan, complete with recipes where relevant (week 2, just cook it all over again!).

This is not a strict regime, merely a guide. You can vary it as you wish, once you have grasped the idea. Variety is the keynote. Make sure you don't eat the same few foods over and over. This risks developing new allergies. It is safer to eat new foods.
Vegetarian dishes are included.

DRINKS

Keep your fluid intake up in whatever way you like. Herb teas are an acquired taste. Try them very weak to start with. Hot water on its own can seem delicious after a few days. We jokingly call this "white tea" (black tea – without the milk; white tea – without the tea either!). It is odd how comforting a warm drink is.

Dilute fruit juices with carbonated spring water and make filtered water ice-cubes; add a slice of apple, a sprig of mint and you have a delicious drink.

SOUPS

Soup daily will fill the gap. Soups can be made in advance and frozen in portions if necessary. They make a good first course for lunch and the evening meal, and are handy to have ready prepared to eat after a busy day before you start to cook for the evening or bathe the baby! Prepare recipes beforehand.

DESSERTS

As such these do not exist on the diet, but by making fruit salads, varying their base daily and using the day's juice, you can make a surprising number of different tastes. Add chopped nuts and dried whole fruits (that you have soaked per instructions).

SPECIAL NOTE FOR CHILDREN

We usually allow rice cakes and special margarine (wheat- and dairy-free). If your child is uncooperative and refuses to eat for the first forty-eight hours, don't worry: hunger will soon be on your side. He or she may be sulking and may indeed be suffering from withdrawal symptoms.

Encourage drinks. Dilute some of the fruit juice and don't worry about cravings for sweets and 'good things. ' By day 3 he or she will be feeling happier.

Once the child realizes there is no alternative, he or she will eat what is prepared. Offer some kind of tangible reward. Children are very good at playing the game when they know the rules.

Puree foods for a small baby, adding a calcium supplement – not soya milk (most baby formulas contain sugar and corn) – and he or she will do fine.

[N.B. Measurements given in these recipes are US equivalents.]

DAY I
Breakfast

SPECIAL SAUSAGE
Fresh minced beef, pork or lamb minced by yourself or the butcher.

Fresh herbs, i.e. sage or mint, chopped sea salt and black pepper to taste.
Potato flour as needed.

Mix first meat, herbs and seasoning together, press into spoon-sized
shapes and roll in potato flour. Alternatively, ask your butcher to make
these. He will if you ask for several lbs. at a time, and then they will be in
sausage skins, which you must then remove. Freeze individually and use
as required. To cook, fry in hot fat.

No supermarket substitutes.

BUBBLE AND SQUEAK
Cooked mashed potato (You can use left-over baked potatoes.)
Cooked green-leaf vegetables (cabbage, kale etc.), chopped
Salt and pepper to taste
Potato flour as needed.

Mix vegetables and seasoning together and either make small portions
by rolling in potato flour or put whole lot in frying pan and keep turning
until brown and crisp. Small portions freeze well.

Soup
FRENCH ONION
1 lb/455 g onions, sliced
1 pint (570 ml or 2 cups) stock (without thickener)
2 tbsp sunflower oil. Salt to taste.
Fry onions in oil until browning. Add stock and simmer for half an hour.

Main Meal
ROAST TURKEY AND VEGETABLES
Roast as much turkey as you like and eat with any vegetables you fancy.
Cook extra potatoes to use for day 2. Use the turkey's giblets to make
gravy and stock for days 2 and 7.

Vegetarian Main Meal
SAVOURY CHESTNUT BAKE

1 onion, peeled and sliced; 1 stick of celery
2 tbsp oil
2 oz/55 g chestnuts, chopped
2 cloves of garlic, peeled
4 oz/115 g walnuts
4 oz/115 g cashews
2 fl oz (60 ml or 1/4 cup) apple juice (more if needed)
6 oz/170 g dried chestnuts, soaked overnight

Drain and simmer with enough water for 2 - 3 hours. Keep water for stock. Salt and pepper to taste.

Set oven at 375°F/195°C. Line a loaf tin with greaseproof paper and brush with oil. Fry onion and celery in oil for 10 minutes. Remove from heat, add to other ingredients and blend in a food processor. Add seasoning, and pile into the baking tin. Cover and bake for 45 minutes. Uncover and bake for an additional 15 minutes.

DAY 2

Breakfast
Use cooked potato from the night before, slice thinly and sprinkle with
sea salt. Quickly fry in a small amount of oil until crisp.

Mushrooms, fried.

Banana slices make a good alternative to mushrooms, but don't overcook
them.

Soup
COURGETTE (ZUCCHINI) SOUP

1 lb/455 g zucchini, chopped
1 ½ pints (850 ml or 3 cups) turkey stock (from giblets of yesterday's
turkey)
Salt and pepper to taste, 1 tsp oil
Lightly fry zucchini in oil and add stock, salt and pepper. Simmer for
half an hour, until the skins are soft. Liquidize. Make double quantities
and freeze for next week.

Main Meal
STIR FRY
1 tbsp oil
Selection of at least 5 vegetables, chopped
Meat of choice (turkey leftovers?)
Salt and pepper to taste
Sweet potato (for side dish)

If possible, pre-heat your oven and put in a sweet potato to cook in its
skin. If you can arrange this, this will be a quick meal.

Pour oil into a heavy-lidded pan or wok. Add vegetables and cover for 3
minutes, shaking while cooking. Add cooked meat, salt and pepper. Cook
for 2-3 minutes.

Serve immediately with sweet potato. For extra flavor add coconut oil to
the sweet potato and sprinkle with powdered cinnamon or nutmeg.

Vegetarian alternative
BEAN LAYER PIE

6 oz/170 g black-eyed peas
Water as needed
1 large onion, chopped
2 tbsp safflower oil
3 medium tomatoes, skinned and chopped
2 sticks of celery, chopped
1 small pepper, seeded and chopped
1 tsp parsley
Salt and pepper
Mashed potatoes

Cook beans in double their volume of water for 30 minutes. Drain. Fry the onion in oil and then add tomato, celery and pepper and cook for about 5 minutes.

Place layers of beans and vegetables in a greased pie pan, adding parsley and seasoning to taste. Cover with mashed potatoes and bake in moderate oven, 275°F/170°C, for 30 minutes. Serve with green vegetables.

NB: Cook double the quantity of potatoes for tomorrow's fish cakes. Put lentils in water to soak overnight for tomorrow's soup.

DAY 3
Breakfast

FISH CAKES
Fish of your choice, cooked
Mashed potato
Salt and pepper to taste
Potato flour as needed
2 tbsp oil
Tomatoes, cooked

Mix together fish, mashed potato and seasoning. Roll mixture in portions in potato flour. Fry in hot oil until brown. Serve with cooked tomato. You can use soft tomatoes to make homemade ketchup by liquefying them in a blender.

Soup
LEEK AND LENTIL SOUP

4 oz/115 g red lentils, soaked overnight; 6 oz/170 g chopped leeks
3 tbsp oil
1 pint (570 ml or 2 cups) vegetable stock
Sea salt
Fresh herbs of your choice

Boil lentils for at least 1 hour. Fry leeks in the oil, in a heavy pan for 10 minutes. Drain lentils, then liquefy in a blender or food processor along with the leeks. Add to vegetable stock and season. Bring to a boil then simmer for 2 minutes. Garnish with chopped herbs.

Main Meal
ROAST DINNER
Use lard, vegetable shortening, or coconut oil for roasting vegetables and basting meat. Keep fat for the next roast and use the meat juices for stock or gravy.

Vegetarian Alternative
STUFFED AUBERGINES (EGGPLANT) (FOR I)

1 aubergine (eggplant)

Oil as needed
1 onion, chopped
2 tomatoes, chopped
¼ lb/340 g mushrooms, chopped; 2 oz/55 g pine nuts
Salt to taste

Halve the aubergine, scoop out the flesh and chop. Heat the oil and fry
the onion until soft. Add aubergine, tomatoes and mushrooms and cook
until soft, but not mushy – about 5 minutes.

Place the aubergine shells in a greased dish, fill with vegetable mixture,
sprinkle on pine nuts and bake in moderate oven for 30 minutes, or
longer, if necessary, at a lower heat. Good with a green salad.

NB: For tomorrow, prepare breakfast by making bacon-mushroom mix.
(Bake potato ahead of time if you like: 1 hour in a 350°F oven.).

DAY 4

Breakfast
BAKED POTATO WITH FILLING
If you haven't pre-baked the potato, do so now. Bake about 1 hour in a
350°F oven. If you've already baked the potato, now preheat the broiler.

4 strips of lean bacon, chopped
4 mushrooms, chopped

Lightly fry bacon, add mushroom, turn off heat and shake in frying pan.
(Reheat mixture if you made it last night.) Use this mixture to fill potato
skin, stirring the mix in with the potato. Pop under the broiler until crisp.

Soup
LIGHT VEGETABLE SOUP
1 tbsp sunflower oil
1 small onion, peeled and finely chopped
6 oz/170 g carrot, cut into 'match sticks' (julienne)
3 sticks celery, sliced
1 ½ pints (850 ml or 2 cups) vegetable stock
Celery leaves
2 tbsp chopped parsley
Black pepper, pinch of salt

Heat oil and fry onion without browning, about 5 minutes. Add carrot
and celery and cook until oil is absorbed. Add stock, bring to a boil and
then simmer for 20 minutes until the vegetable is tender, but not mushy.

Main Meal
RATATOUILLE

1 tbsp oil
1 large onion, peeled and chopped
1 large aubergine (eggplant), cut into 1-inch cubes
3 small zucchini, sliced
1 green pepper, seeded and diced
1 red pepper, seeded and diced
10 oz/285 g tomatoes, skinned (dropped into boiling water for 2 minutes
to help separate the skins) and chopped

1 tbsp fresh basil leaves (chopped)
Salt and pepper to taste

Fry the onion for 10 minutes and then add all the other ingredients. Cook, covered, for 15 minutes, stirring frequently. Can be frozen.

Vegetarian Alternative
BAKED POTATO WITH HAZELNUT SAUCE (SERVES 4)
1 large potato with skin (side dish)
1 tbsp oil
1 onion, peeled and chopped
1 tbsp hazelnut butter
4 oz/115 g chopped roast hazelnuts (roast under grill)
½ lb/225 g tomatoes, chopped and skinned (see above)
Salt and pepper to taste
Cauliflower, broken into florets and steamed till tender

Have potato baking in oven (about 350°F) for at least 1 hour.
Fry onion, then add all other ingredients except for the cauliflower. Season and pour mixture over cauliflower. Serve piping hot with baked potato.

Y 5

Breakfast
Try grilled fish
Squeezed fruit or vegetable juice

Soup
LEEK AND POTATO SOUP

1 tbsp sunflower oil
1 small onion, peeled and sliced
1 large (8 oz/225 g) leek, washed and sliced
12 oz/340 g potatoes, peeled and cut into 1/4-inch cubes
1 ½ pints (850 ml or 3 cups) homemade vegetable stock
Bay leaf
Salt and pepper

Heat oil and fry onion for 3-4 minutes. Add the leek and potatoes and
stir well. Leave on a low heat for a few minutes, covered, until oil is
absorbed. Add stock, bay leaf and plenty of black pepper. Cover, bring
to a boil and then simmer for 15 minutes. Remove bay leaf and serve
piping hot.

Main Meal
BEEF PATTIES

2 medium onions, finely chopped
1 lb minced (or ground) beef
Salt and pepper, potato flour
Sunflower oil

Put onions, beef and seasoning into the food processor and blend on a
low setting. Make ¼ lb/(115 g) portions of meat mixture for each patty,
roll in potato flour and flatten. Cook in hot oil for 5 minutes each side,
making sure each patty is well cooked through.

Vegetarian Alternative
 MILLET AND COURGETTE RISOTTO

2 tbsp oil
2 onions, peeled and chopped
1 red pepper, chopped and seeded; 1 (16 oz/455 g) zucchini, sliced
2 cloves of garlic, finely chopped; 8 oz/225 g millet
1 pint (570 ml/2 cups) water
Salt and pepper

Fry onions, red pepper, zucchini and garlic in a saucepan for 10 minutes.
Add millet and water and bring to a boil. Cover and turn down the heat;
cook for 20 minutes, until the millet is cooked and fluffy. Season. Serve
with crispy lettuce.

NB: For tomorrow, put the lentils in pan of water to soak overnight.
Make the gazpacho if you have time and leave it in the fridge.

DAY 6

Breakfast
Fruit bowl

Soup
GAZPACHO

1 medium onion, skinned and chopped
2 tbsp oil
1 small green pepper, chopped and seeded
½ pint (285 ml/1 cup) tomato puree (blended, skinned tomatoes)
I clove garlic crushed (optional)
Small quantity other vegetables at hand, e.g. zucchini
Seasoning
Watercress
5 oz/140 g cucumber, chopped

Sauté onion in oil for 5 minutes. Add other ingredients except seasoning, watercress and cucumber. Simmer for 15-20 minutes, season and chill. Serve garnished with watercress and with chopped cucumber on the side to use as croutons.

Main Meal
MARRAKECH CHICKEN AND LENTILS

1 tbsp. 100% pure virgin coconut oil
4 skinless chicken breasts chopped into pieces
6 oz potato, buckwheat or any other grain-free flour
8 oz brown lentils, rinsed and picked over
12 whole dried apricots (3 oz.), quartered
2 oz fresh parsley, chopped
½ tsp. fresh ginger, chopped
½ tsp. salt, or to taste
1/4 tsp. *EACH ground allspice, cinnamon, cumin and red pepper (cayenne)*
120 ml water with 1 teaspoon of vegetable bouillon powder dissolved into it.

Heat oven to 350°F/175C. Heat the coconut oil in a frying pan. Coat the chicken pieces with flour, shaking off excess. Add to frying pan and cook until lightly browned, about 5 minutes. Remove and place on a plate.

Add lentils, spring onions, apricots, raisins, parsley, ginger, salt and spices to frying pan. Cook, stirring, for 1 minute.

Transfer to an ovenproof dish. Put the chicken on top. Add water, cover and place in oven. Bake 30 minutes, uncover and bake 20 minutes longer or until chicken and lentils are tender.
Serves 4

Vegetarian Alternative
ITALIAN LENTIL CASSEROLE

12 oz/340 g green lentils (soaked overnight)
2 pints (21.14 litres or 4 cups) water
2 tbsp oil
1 onion, skinned and chopped
6 oz/170 g mushrooms, chopped
1 lb/455 g tomatoes, chopped
Clove of garlic, crushed
1 tsp fresh marjoram, oregano or basil (but any other herb will do)
Salt and pepper

Boil lentils in water for 35-40 minutes. Drain. Heat oil and fry onion, then the other vegetables; cook for 5 minutes. Grease casserole, add lentils to the vegetable mixture, add herbs and seasoning to taste and bake for half an hour at 325°F/180°C.

Keep 2 tablespoons of tomato puree for tomorrow's paella.

DAY 7

Breakfast

Buckwheat pancakes with *real* maple syrup
Use graham flour or egg replacer to make it stick together.
Add blueberries or other fruit filler as desired.

Soup
CARROT SOUP

2 pints (4 cups) turkey stock
1 lb/455 g carrots, chopped
3 large leeks (or 1 large onion), chopped
Parsley, chopped

Put all ingredients except parsley into a pan and simmer until the vegetables are soft. Liquefy in a blender or food processor and return to heat. Serve garnished with parsley. If you want to, you can leave vegetables in whole pieces for a luncheon-type soup.

Main Meal
HAM AND VEGETABLES

Joint of ham
Water to cover
½ pint (285 ml/1 1/3 cups) pineapple juice
Potatoes with skin on
Carrots, chopped
Salt and pepper to taste

Soak ham joint for 2 hours (shoulder is an inexpensive cut). Put the joint in a pan and bring to a boil, then pour off the water and cut off the rind. Put the joint into a roasting tin or oven-proof dish. Baste with pineapple juice and roast at 325°F/180°C for 30 minutes, or until fat is brown.

Bake potatoes in the oven. Use skewers through each to shorten cooking time. Carrots can be put in a covered casserole with some water and seasoning and baked along with the potatoes in a low oven for 2 hours, a hotter oven for 1 to 1 ½ hours.

NB: For tomorrow, cook enough ham to have cold, plus extra potato for bubble and squeak (back to Day I).

Vegetarian Alternative
FISH-FREE PAELLA

Sunflower oil
3 oz/85 p mushrooms sliced
5 oz/140 g quinoa, uncooked (alternatively use buckwheat pasta)
½ pint (285 ml/1 cups) pineapple juice
½ pint (285 ml/1 cups) water
2 tbsp tomato puree
2 oz/55 g sultanas (raisins)
½ small green pepper, chopped
2 oz/55 g nuts
Pineapple rings to garnish

Sauté the sliced mushrooms in the sunflower oil in a large pan. Add the rice and cook for a few minutes. Add juice, water and tomato puree. Simmer for about 25-30 minutes until the liquid is absorbed and rice is tender. Add sultanas, green pepper and coarsely chopped or grated nuts. Heat through and serve with pineapple rings.

Appendix D

Lowering your pesticides intake from food

As I explained in Chapter 17, it is not always practical or economical to follow a strictly organic diet. In any case you run the risk of being cheated by dishonest food vendors. The official goalposts are often being changed, for the benefit of the industry, of course, not for the benefit of the wary consumer.

But you can still dramatically lower your family's exposure to chemical pesticides by choosing the least pesticide-contaminated fruits and vegetables with the aid of the Environmental Working Group's *Shopper's Guide to Pesticides in Produce*.

The *Shopper's Guide* is a handy, wallet-size card that lists the "Dirty Dozen" most contaminated fruits and vegetables, as well as the twelve most "Consistently Clean" items. It's available for free download at www. foodnews.org. The newest edition of the *Guide* comes in both English and Spanish versions.

The *Shopper's Guide* was based on the results of nearly 43,000 tests for pesticides on produce by the Department of Agriculture and the Food and Drug Administration between 2000 and 2004. EWG's computer analysis found that consumers could cut their pesticide exposure by almost ninety percent by avoiding the most contaminated fruits and vegetables and eating the least contaminated instead.

Eating the twelve most contaminated fruits and vegetables will expose a person to about fifteen pesticides a day, on average. Eating the twelve least contaminated will expose a person to fewer than two pesticides a day.

"Federal produce tests tell us that some fruits and vegetables are so likely to be contaminated with pesticides that you should always buy them organic," said Richard Wiles, EWG's senior vice president. "Others are so consistently clean that you can eat them with less concern. With the *Shopper's Guide* in your pocket, it's easy to tell which is which."

EWG's analysis of federal testing data found the following:

Peaches and apples topped the Dirty Dozen list. Almost ninety-seven percent of peaches tested positive for pesticides, and almost eighty-seven percent had two or more pesticide residues. About ninety-two percent of apples tested positive, and seventy-nine percent had two or more pesticides.

Onions, avocados, and sweet corn headed the Consistently Clean list. For all three foods, more than ninety percent of the samples tested had no detectable pesticide residues. Here are the full 2006 lists:

The "Dirty Dozen" (starting with the worst)

- peaches
- apples
- sweet bell peppers
- celery
- nectarines
- strawberries
- cherries
- pears
- grapes (imported)
- spinach
- lettuce
- potatoes

The "Cleanest 12" (starting with the best)

- onions
- avocados
- sweet corn (frozen)
- pineapples

- mangoes

- asparagus

- sweet peas (frozen)

- kiwi fruit

- bananas

- cabbage

- broccoli

- papaya

Because the toxic effects of pesticides are worrisome, not well understood, or in some cases completely unstudied, shoppers are wise to minimize exposure to pesticides whenever possible.

While washing and rinsing fresh produce can reduce levels of some pesticides, it does not eliminate them. Peeling also reduces exposures, but valuable nutrients often go down the drain with the peel. The best option is to eat a varied diet, wash all produce, and choose organic when possible to reduce exposure to potentially harmful chemicals.

Although the *EWG Shopper's Guide* only measures pesticide residues on produce, buying organic also makes sense if you're concerned about bacterial contamination. Organic farmers meet all the sanitation standards required of conventional growers and, on, top of that, meet tight restrictions on the use of compost and other organic material that do not apply to conventional fruit and vegetable growers.

[quoted with permission]
The Environmental Working Group is a nonprofit research organization based in Washington, DC that uses the power of information to protect human health and the environment. The Group's research on food safety is viewable online at www.ewg.org/ issues/siteindex/issues.php?issueid=3004.

APPENDIX E SOME USEFUL ADDRESSES

Here are some useful contact addresses to get you started. However in these days of Google and the Internet, no-one need get stuck for contacts. If you feel you have a site which would be helpful to sufferes of food allergy and genetic food intolerance and would like it listed here in future editions, please contact me at:

Dr Keith Scott-Mumby
PO Box 816,
Palm Springs,
CA 92263-0816
(USA)

Here you will find US doctors who practice alternative allergy medicine of the kind you have been reading about:

American Academy of Environmental Medicine
7701 E Kellogg Dr Suite 625
Wichita, KS 67207-1705
Phone: (316) 684-5500
www.aaem.com/

Here is the British equivalent:

British Society of Allergy, Environmental and Nutritional Medicine,
PO Box 7,
Knighton
Tel: 01547 550380,
Fax: 01547 550339
www.minotaur.org.uk

This association of doctors are all very inclined to alternative medicine solutions for health but not necessarily well-versed in allergies:

American College for the Advancement of Medicine
24411 Ridge Route Suite 115
Laguna Hills,
CA 92653
949 309 3520
www.acam.org

Allergy Testing, cytotoxic blood tests

ALCAT test
Cell Science Systems
1239 East Newport Center Drive, Suite 101
Deerfield Beach, FL 33442
Phone: (800) US ALCAT (872-5228)
Phone: (954) 426-2304
E-mail: info@alcat.com

Nutron test (now called the Novo test), available through the following centers:

Cherokee Family Medical Centre
9766 Highway 92 Suite 200
Woodstock
GA 30188
Tel:(1) 770 926 8717
E-mail: drjlw@flash.net

Dr Robert J Bos
178 East 85th Street
New York, NY 10028
Tel:(1) 212 861 2081
E-mail: consult@drbos.com

Allergy Support Groups

Beware of those funded and run (secretly) by pharmaceutical firms with a drug agenda.

Kids with Food Allergies
73 Old Dublin Pike, Ste 10, #163
Doylestown, PA 18901
(215) 230-5394
www.kidswithfoodallergies.org

Great support group started by America Nathan-Hill nearly 30 years ago:

Action Against Allergy,
PO Box 279,
Twickenham, TW1 4QQ,
Tel: 0208 8892 2711 Fax: 0208 892 4950

Foresight, (the association for pre-conceptual care),
28 The Paddock,
Godalming,
Surrey GU7 1KD
UK
Tel: 01483 427839
www.surreyweb.net

Hyperactive Childrens' Support Group,
71 Whyke Lane,
Chichester,
West Sussex, PO19 2LD

Alternative Health Laboratories

Institute of Parasitic Diseases
Diagnostic Laboratory
3530 E. Indian School Road, Suite 3
Phoenix, Arizona 85018
602-955-4211

Genova Diagnostics
63 Zillicoa Street
Asheville, NC 28801
USA
Telephone: (828)253-0621
www.gdx.net/home/

Medical Diagnostic Laboratory
3250 Westchester Ave.
Bronx, New York 10461
212-828-1500

Organic Foods Standards

The full set of regulations contained in the National Standards on Organic Agricultural Production and Handling can be viewed or downloaded from the USDA at:
http://www.ams.usda.gov/nop/nop2000/Final%20Rule/nopfinal.pdf

Organic Suppliers Directory
In depth news, information, direction, research and data resources to all segments of the organic and natural product industries. Includes a directory of suppliers.
http://www.naturalfoodnet.com/nfnportal

Henry Doubleday Research Organization
A British organisation, registered charity, world-leading organization dedicated to researching and promoting organic gardening, farming and food.
Ryton Organic Gardens
Coventry
Warwickshire
United Kingdom
CV8 3LG
Tel: +44 (0) 24 7630 3517
Email: enquiry@hdra.org.uk
www.gardenorganic.org.uk

Nutrition Organizations And Foundations

Price-Pottenger Nutrition Foundation
7890 Broadway
Lemon Grove, CA 91945
800-366-3748 (in the US) or (619) 462-7600
www.price-pottenger.org/index.htm
info@price-pottenger.org

The Weston A. Price Foundation
PMB 106-380, 4200 Wisconsin Ave., NW, Washington DC 20016
Phone: (202) 363-4394 | Fax: (202) 363-4396
www.westonaprice.org

The McCarrison Society
179 Friern Road
London
SE22 0BD
Tel: +44(0)20 7133 2440
http://www.mccarrisonsociety.org.uk/
info@mccarrisonsociety.org.uk

and much more commercial than the other organizations in this section:

Institute of Optimum Nutrition,
13 Blades Court,
Deodar Road,
London SW15 2NU
Tel: 020 8877 9993
www.ion.ac.uk

Index

E

tartaric acid 253
Tempeh 261
The American College of Asthma, Allergy, & Immunology 189
The Hydrogen Breath Test 253
The Moldy Patient 256
The 'problem patient' 251
therapeutic diagnosis 163
thyroid 18, 109, 149
Thyroid disease 149
Tinea 256
Touch for Health 230
treats 165, 177, 181, 213, 234
turkey-tail mushroom 257

U

ulcers 69
universal reactors 161
Urticaria 145
urticaria 90, 206, 209

V

Vegetarian 275, 278, 280, 281, 284, 286, 288, 290
vegetarians 57, 141, 142, 197, 198, 199, 217
violent behavior 73
viruses 252
Vitamin allergy 111
vitamin and mineral supplements 135, 147, 150
vitiated food 53

W

Wheat Contacts 267
wheal 225, 226
Wheat-free bread 219
Withdrawal symptoms 121, 154
withdrawal symptoms 60, 151, 154, 176, 200, 276
woolly brain 14, 62, 77

X

xylitol 256

Y

Yeast and mold 219
yeast and mold 92, 145, 219

Z